Introduction

Welcome to a book about the modern-day American vaccine marketplace. The drug marketplace where our government suggests love and care in addressing our infectious disease fears. Our government compels citizens to fear infectious diseases and seeks love for authorities that offer a protective remedy using hurried science to deliver a drug from a vaccine industry it controls and promotes as a solution to the current infectious disease crisis. Our government promotes vaccines as the past and future great protective drugs for our citizens during a moment of crisis. But does not inform citizens of a scandalous side of vaccines, the Vaccine Law and the government's promotional public policy. An ongoing law and policy most citizens do not understand. Our government unwaveringly encourages citizens to embrace vaccines as the best public health strategy for infectious diseases, not to seek answers and understanding.

As you may guess from the book title, this book takes a slightly different approach to evaluating vaccines. In this book, I hope to assess the state of vaccines, vaccine management, and the poorly understood vaccine programs suggested by our government as being the path to a safe and well-informed citizenry. Our government promotes vaccines above all other infectious disease treatments, often using limited science and suggestions that they will use good manufacturing practices and research standards to address an ongoing standard for developing safe vaccines. And we will look briefly at the COVID-19 infectious outbreak and vaccine, and what it may mean to you, not just as the reader, but you and your family. Is there an easy path to a safe and effective COVID-19 vaccine? A vaccine that will suggestively deliver protection from the infectious disease and promises to cause limited or no serious adverse vaccine reactions. These are important questions citizens often ask many parties that oversee vaccine development and public health. Is our government trustworthy to deliver a safe and effective vaccine, as they function as the primary vaccine researcher and developer, promotor, advocate, and of course most importantly as the sole protector of the next novel vaccine and any related cost of liability to all citizens? Do citizens understand a conflicting commercial quasi-government entity really serves as the answer our government offers citizens for a safe vaccine for all citizens.

We are told by our government a safe COVID-19 vaccine will be here at warp speed. And if all citizens get vaccinated, we will all be protected from the horrible infectious disease and the spiraling economic collateral damage it causes. The government, the media, and multiple parties endorse a suggestive path for vaccines to provide public protection, if only we follow their direction and instruction. The message of love and fear and a twist on science offer citizens science and drug information few citizens seek to understand, as the fear of an infectious pandemic running wild surely exceeds the fear of a new vaccine and any potentially bad adverse drug reactions such a rushed vaccine may cause. Hopefully, the vaccine does what our government promises the vaccine should do, by providing a protective barrier to the spread of the infection, rather than cause serious medical complications few scientists will understand, which could be called the weakest link to developing a safe vaccine and a secure wall against infectious disease containment.

Citizens should open their minds to understand the current state of the vaccine ecosystem. An avaricious underworld of vaccine interests where authorities and vaccine manufacturers work hand-in-hand to ensure the protection of vaccine manufacturing, research, and development. Citizens should consider protection and development of a safe vaccine drug essential, but safety concerns are mostly an afterthought to most vaccine-related parties. The primary concern of promoting protection is competing in an open drug development race to save humanity. This protective disease management business strategy is suggestively corrupt as the race to understand and control infectious diseases has been going on since the beginning of humanity. Highly intelligent people offer citizens facts and evidence today that suggest a sound and understood vaccine science but will totally fail to document and evaluate vaccine-related injuries and adverse events. And will seek to shift fear away from our flawed and dysfunctional healthcare systems by promoting a system of medicines few understand or even care to understand. As fear that a vaccine-related injury may occur is considered small and widely propagandized as barely a concern at all. Citizens should not be concerned with libelous actions caused by vaccines as our government offers a false and flawed safety net to protect its citizens. "Fear the infectious disease most", authorities will shout, not the vaccine-related injuries, for the infectious disease is much more dangerous. Trust authorities to deliver protection and safety, as it is in their interest to protect all citizens, which I hope to show is a false promise.

As the author, I have little interest in advancing philosophical or political motivated beliefs or opinions about vaccines. The idea of false opinions and beliefs are troubling to citizens where mechanisms for vaccine injuries are poorly understood.

Tangential arguments and narratives in politics and law can be made to fit a preferred view of vaccine science favored by some parties, but I prefer to stick with basic drug science which is learned and discovered in scientific research and documented in scientific literature. Science and politics do not always blend well, as our politicians often provide no documented science to support their preferred scientific narrative. But where would we be as a democracy without science? Science is the foundation of creativity and human discovery, and the basis for a substantial portion of our economy. Living in a democracy without understood science is unfathomable, as scientists would be required to follow a false set of facts and work with medical practitioners that are dishonest and untruthful, which is what was once the standards of science and medicine centuries ago. Should we go back?

Infectious diseases again have been around for ages, while vaccines are both an old and a new breed of prescription drugs. The idea one would develop a natural protective immunity through contracting an infectious disease and recovering was recognized long ago as a protective acquired form of immunity against future infections of the same diseases, but the concept of isolating noninvasive antigens as a method for vaccination was discovered only a few centuries ago. The protective immunity developed using vaccines is a limited form of protection against the infectious diseases often caused by pathogens that cause serious infectious disease outbreaks. Large sections of the population may die from such outbreaks, and a cure, any suggested cure may be worth trying if the number of deaths is exceedingly high. Who would want widespread suffering and death, over a few adverse treatment complications some might ask? Not much of the population when offered the choice, but perhaps more citizens would ask more questions when given full disclosure of safety and liability concerns that are poorly addressed, or if the infectious outbreak does not impact all citizens.

Vaccines were a great scientific discovery, a protective drug which aids the body in developing protective antibodies using a normal immune system process. Vaccines emerged from a long observed protective immunity practice, and was first documented as an observed scientific drug-related protocol which took centuries to evolve as an understood protective drug mechanism in an immune system that scientists did not know much about or how the immune system worked. The general concept of how vaccines work is understood that vaccines produced protective immunity through the development of antibodies, but also unfortunately can cause adverse vaccine reactions which are often omitted from medical discussions. The early lessons of adverse vaccine reactions from the earliest vaccines was that whatever was going on inside the body would clear up and go away. The common implied understanding being vaccines are mostly a safe drug option, especially when compared to death and serious infectious disease complications, which in the early years of vaccine use had no other treatment options. Vaccines were the sole option for protection from infectious disease for more than a century.

As vaccines evolved and many diseases began being treated with vaccines, government authorities with little understanding of the science began to preach to the citizens who likewise lacked an understanding and accepted whatever they were told to believe. More infectious outbreaks continued to evolve, and antibiotics had not yet been discovered. The value of vaccines held their ground but fell down several notches when the discovery of penicillin and other antibiotics took off as many diseases became easily treatable with antibiotics. Government authorities, however, continued to value vaccines as a protective infectious medicine, but public sentiment grew hostile and several adverse vaccine concerns involving several vaccines became problems that required attention and demanded vaccine safety concerns must be addressed.

The science relating to vaccine use show vaccines have a functional purpose, but our government's authorities have routinely ignored safety concerns and serious adverse events that occur following a vaccine administration. Drug safety and efficacy issues became key topics on the way to legislating the Food, Drug and Cosmetics Act which was enacted in 1938. Beginning a path to ensuring all drugs are safe and effective as promised by manufacturers and all parties prescribing and selling drugs, and shifted the Food and Drug Administration (FDA) from a backburner federal agency forward to being the highest authority on drugs in our nation. Efficacy (also called effectiveness) of the drugs were put at the forefront, while drug safety was a secondary issue of lesser importance for decades. Science and medical clinical observations and drug applications, often physician observed adverse reactions, were limiting factors to observation of drug adverse concerns. It took decades, but eventually the government added layers of safety measures on many drug classes, creating specialized classifications for many drugs, including controlled substances and the government added layers of regulatory law enforcement to address these drug safety concerns.

Vaccine safety concerns remained somewhat stable in this era of newfound drug regulation, but vaccine safety was still a concern among many medical professionals and citizens, even as new vaccines were discovered including oral versions, which were breakthroughs. But while vaccines developed a track record of effectiveness during this time where our government was shifting to promoting drug safety, vaccines never fully developed a track record of logging and addressing vaccine safety concerns. In fact, the vaccine safety reporting and science behind vaccine injuries track record was exceedingly poor. Where the government and doctors revered a single dose of medicine for infectious disease protection, the public often complained of minor and serious adverse drug reactions, which were generally dismissed as lacking significance to doctors and government drug regulators and authorities.

Whereas vaccine safety was put on the backburner with poor recordkeeping and limited pharmacovigilant research and reporting (deeper drug action studies), the adverse complications related to Swine flu vaccines became a public health fiasco in 1976, as an outbreak of Swine Flu led to a vaccine that would cause a serious medical condition known as Guillain-Barre Syndrome. Vaccine safety and vaccine efficacy hit a wall, and the resulting injury concerns changed vaccines and the public perception of vaccines going forward. The public image for vaccines had to be changed and suggestively fixed. Perhaps the vaccine manufacturers could not make the vaccines safe, but the government could make the public believe they are safe, by actively promoting the protective actions of vaccines as being the most vital function of the drug's actions and suggesting the government would cover all vaccine-related injuries with fair compensation provided to the vaccine-injured patients.

Vaccine safety however became a key sticking point for doctors, manufacturers, and our government's Department of Justice (also known as the DOJ), as manufacturers could not guarantee safety and fewer adverse vaccine reactions. In fact, the vaccine-related injury track record for many vaccines became well-founded public health safety concerns. All drug laws mandate drugs, including vaccines, must be documented as being both safe (listing warnings, precautions and known adverse reactions) and effective (listing approved use and proper dosing). Doctors, pharmacists, and regulators have both a professional and legal obligations and duties to address these specific drug concerns. Vaccine safety concerns however became a philosophical legal matter, as the government stepped in and decided to reclassify vaccines. All parties of government, all three branches of government (Legislative, Executive and Judicial) prominently included in the discussions and decisions, declared vaccines a special and exclusive class of drugs, which would be afforded special privileges. These special privileges continue today and establish vaccines as having rare exclusivity never seen before in the history of drugs, and surely not in modern drug history relating to drug safety and public health matters.

I will cover these details more in the book, but readers should understand these concerns are valid medical concerns and are understood as both philosophical and scientific concerns. Do citizens understand the safety risks related to vaccines, which are detectable adverse events, and not just a narrow group of vaccine-related injuries promoted by government agencies? Or that vaccine risks are minimalized to offset a promotional viewpoint our government has prearranged as part of its duty in developing and advocating vaccines as the suggested preferred infectious class medicine. These poorly understood promoted public-viewpoint statements were adopted to provide the greatest level of arrogance to our government and to permit aggressive vaccine endorsement through a few authorities and legal professionals which was adopted into law in 1986, and has grown since with overconfidence in-house within our government as its established promotional vaccine messages, and acts today as entry-level messages stated by our vaccine industry advertisers. Today, vaccines are one of the most dynamic pharmaceutical research and development institutional industries in existence, with exceedingly limited oversight and wide discretionary drug research practices. Shameful practices really, but I will let you be the judge.

Detailed investigation of vaccine-related injuries has not however kept pace with the promotional public messages made by our government since 1986. Authorities have failed to fulfill its promise to address vaccine safety in a fair and just manner since granting liability protections to vaccine manufacturers and medical professionals. These vaccine injury concerns are critical issues that are overlooked as they relate to drug safety in general. As the government has sunken hundreds of billions of dollars into vaccine research, development, regulation, promotion, advocacy, legislation, and other actions since the National Childhood Vaccine Injury Act of 1986 (which is commonly referred to as the Vaccine Act, the NCVIA, or simply the Vaccine Law) was enacted. In fact, the government will without hesitation claim billions of dollars have been granted to injured parties, through a vaccine injury program called the Vaccine Injury Compensation Program (commonly referred to in legal circles and throughout this book as the VICP), as a unique creation only our government lawyers and politicians could possibly come up with as a creative and disgusting legal resolution created as the sole answer to address a threat by manufacturers to pull vaccines from the American marketplace. In return for legal liability protection, vaccine injury compensation settlement claims were promised as a government resolution to cover all individuals injured by vaccine-related adverse reactions. Politicians and lawyers even using children as a public selling point to gain public support leverage for a legislated action to protect vaccine manufacturers, if anyone cares to make note of the suggestive use of "Childhood" injuries in name selected for the Vaccine Act.

Again, I will get into details later, but the VICP is perhaps one of the most evil, divisive government promises ever made to citizens, which is saying a lot considering our government's, and other governments' track record, with at least a dozen injustices coming to mind instantly, and apologies to all citizens that have suffered from these awful government injustices and actions over many decades and centuries. The path our government has taken with its vaccine promises are mostly fabricated and created to get a law enacted that is both harmful and wrong to individual citizens. Society has not benefitted from greatly accelerated safe vaccine developments, but has become part of a grand science experiment, with many implied benefits and suggestive therapeutic uses in addition to the infectious disease protective uses once suggested as their primary purpose. Vaccines continue to have many adverse drug-related complications. Maybe the public has not heard of these complications, as pharmaceutical companies have moved much of the research and clinical testing overseas, where less oversight is both favorable and welcoming, and the test populations are large. And the FDA approval process has become much more favorable to global pharmaceutical developments with lagging reporting and safety concerns, which were promised in early drug laws that such safety evaluations would be prompt and rigorous, but suddenly reporting of adverse drug events now take decades to address as reported drug safety concerns. Who is running the FDA ship? Is it the Admiral with unfettered authority? As in the old days of admiralty law, where the captain rules the ship, everyone else get off the ship if you do not like how the ship is being run. All American citizens please report to the deck to exit the government's disastrous vaccine ship.

The immediate needs of "society" and specialized groups of citizens, including political interest groups and pharmaceutical manufacturers, play vital roles in underwriting drug safety regulation. It is a public health concern and a medical concern. You may ask are these concerns not the same? Well, these concerns are not the same but are entwined government actions and a broad suggested concern for public safety and drug safety. In fact, law enforcement has been enjoined to the cause with greater granted power to impose punishment to citizens in recent decades. Who decides what these important new causes and actions are in the name of citizens? Government authorities and elected officials make most of these decisions and suggest honest and wholesome attempts at addressing all drug and public health concerns; but most of these authorities are not scientists and rarely have a clue as to how the medical professions operate and practice. Again, the ship is a mess, and the captain is drinking too much.

The issue of addressing public safety, like the current pandemic and drug safety laws, have gone on for thousands of years. The seriousness of the current COVID-19 virus pandemic is not without concern personally or professionally, but it is not as concerning as other risks and concerns we should address as a society. COVID-19 mortality rates are significant but has only a slightly higher mortality death rate as noted during other cyclical viral and bacterial outbreaks. Public actions of isolating or quarantine and face covering have slowed the virus spread, but certainly will not be the factors that will end the spread of the infectious disease. As the end of the outbreak is uncertain, society is dealing with a novel virus with unknown predictive factors of spread and mortality and many other uncertainties that suggest a major change in many societies and economies worldwide. Our society scrambles and cannot stay static but demands changes to rectify flaws in our governance. A government that does not seem capable of addressing an infectious outbreak and a government that imposes economic chaos to address infectious outbreaks.

The COVID-19 outbreak is a pandemic by scientific definitions, but where does it measure up against past outbreaks? And is it driven by public mania and political mania to stir a mad scramble to gain public empathy and concern? Or is it a momentous scientific scramble by medical professionals looking to address a shortage in resources and supplies along with insufficient training on what public health concerns must be discussed? Who should we trust for our society's protection and survival? Can we trust the authorities' plans and schemes to find answers for a better tomorrow? I suggest we use extreme caution and evaluate facts as related to understood and well-defined science. Our government will suggest it is doing so on our behalf yet fails in what appears to be another government-provoked economic and medical catastrophe.

My concerns for drug facts are also the concerns of many scientists and medical professionals and are related to concerns linking all infectious disease outbreaks and vaccine safety fears to citizens who simply demand drug facts be addressed. As citizens are the final healthcare and drug decision-makers in our society, not authoritarian leaders. Science is science, and the facts are understood laws of nature discovered in science. Politics and the laws of society are often less certain when chaos arises from political actions based on biased authoritative opinions and beliefs. Do we as citizens accept the laws of select authorities' personal beliefs over the laws of science? Or do we as citizens require laws of nature be understood and pursued, and mandate our government enact laws that comply with natural science, and not some authority's arbitrary opinions of science or sentiment of the few we grant as being in a position to make decisions which are not correct and can be harmful to many citizens.

These conflicts and battles over enacted laws are not new and have gone on for centuries. Authorities have always dictated the rules of law to fit their self-interests, often skipping over laws of nature and science, and are often laws that favor their self-interests. Many leaders have historically created a need for logical-thought professions to manipulate political views to fit their preferred narrative, and these beliefs and opinions are given justification and enacted as laws. Lawyers and legal scholars argue points of law, thought to be logical, but often fail to understand the source of the science. It is a common problem in interpreting a law, lawyers do not care to understand the science, and doctors do not care to understand the law, as being suggestive of reaching some mutually beneficial compromised logical deduction of truth, which often leads to misunderstandings and poorly applied discretionary decisions. I have heard it argued many times and would argue a law is not much of a law unless citizens fully understand the law. And if both citizens and licensed professionals, like doctors and pharmacists, do not understand the drug or medical law, an enacted law is mostly garbage. Most citizens fail to understand pharmacists have far more knowledge of drug laws than most citizens including lawyers, whereas medical laws often act as discretionary compendiums to physicians to make clinical decisions and as guides for safe practice standards. Vaccine laws are from a different planet. Most likely because they were created by lawyers and political advocates from a different planet.

It is clear from history, citizens and authorities in general do not understand the natural sciences well, and that infectious outbreaks cause significant economic and collateral damages fully related to the outbreak and political decisions made in the name of public health interests. Infectious diseases are not one-time events but are repeating events which must be reconciled and addressed for current and future safety of all citizens. Should we shelter in place and hope for a medical miracle? Or hope a woefully underfunded medical system and poorly resourced government will band together and serve all citizens? Vaccines are not the perfect solution to address infectious outbreak problems but are promoted by authorities as the current "best" option, which are sometimes a moon-shot type of discovery, or better yet a Mars-shot. What could go wrong? We have great scientists and great allies. Hopefully, one of them can discover the first great safe viral-sourced vaccine since that has not really been done before since the discovery of vaccines. Or a vaccine may become one of the epic vaccine-related injury problems related to an infectious outbreak. As vaccine safety could be, as it often is, overlooked as it relates to a complex adverse medical complication few medical professionals are prepared to address and are often referred to as unforeseen complications. The pilot sees the coming storm and bravely flies right into the major storm telling everyone aboard there are no problems to be concerned about, we have a good plane to fly, and the storm appears manageable. Wow, the passenger, citizens, should feel safer already.

My first professional thoughts are I hope all medical professionals are fully trained and have experienced and learned the wildly unpredictable adverse vaccine reaction injuries that vaccines can cause before setting out to practice and prescribe vaccines as their answer to an infectious outbreak. But I know, most medical professionals have limited vaccine knowledge and training but jump right into the fight with bravado and stupidity, with a hint of possibility for luck in addressing the infectious pathogen. This is what our government and medical professionals have been living off for decades, as the government has been consistently been making promises, then changing the rules and promised solutions. As experts and scientists continue to research novel and understood vaccine mechanisms of action, they often do not address adverse complications which are vital to making an informed medical judgement call. The government has created and enacted solutions for addressing the legal issue related to vaccine liability but has never had any solution for making the vaccines safer or making vaccine safety data more accessible to the public or to medical professionals.

All drug regulators and scientists know vaccines are imperfect drugs and all vaccines cause drug-related injuries, but most do not understand the depth of actions taken to marginalize the safety profiles of select vaccines determined by select authorities as being vital to the public. A broad promotional narrative is used to imply that vaccines are valuable, and vaccines do work as suggestive protection, but also make efforts to marginalize adverse vaccine-related injury concerns. Authorities dismiss observed science as concerns until they understand the causational vaccine injury mechanisms, which are given discretion to cause harm by select authorities to random individuals. Since 1986, authorities have been making the final decision for citizens even as it is mandatory the individual citizens have the right to have access to information to make informed decisions based on observed and understood science causing many adverse drug events.

Citizens face critical decisions every day including issues relating to personal finance, day-to-day living, and for many citizens important concerns relating to individual healthcare choices. It is vital we understand COVID-19 and many other novel infectious disease viruses will over time spread through society and will be around for the foreseeable future. It is better we learn the steps we must take now to prepare for such infectious outbreaks, and to prepare for future pandemics. The world will never be completely free of infectious diseases. But are vaccines the safest drug option to be the answer to infectious diseases, and does our government really offer a safety net for injuries triggered by vaccines. Vaccines are a present-day part of a scientific movement to address future diseases and current diseases by using vaccines which offer limited legal recourse for citizens. Will vaccines also cure cancer, influenza, COVID, bacterial infections, cavities, and be accepted for use in other novel therapeutic treatment protocols? Maybe vaccines will one day be useful as a drug of first choice in a wide-range of treatment protocols, or more likely could become drugs of last resort as the safety concerns may never be fully addressed. Authorities often employ grade school-level drug scientific uncertainty choices in promoting vaccines, where they know a vaccine can cause harmful drug injuries but take little action. Why? Because our government has told citizens they would take care of the vaccine injury problems as they arise. Yet, as the problems arise both nonscientific and scientific authorities fail in their duty to address adverse vaccine and drug related injuries, known in medical circles as Adverse Drug Reactions (ADRs), which has resulted in the massive legislative failure to address ADRs by granting authorities broad discretion and allowing suggestive "good faith efforts" as being adequate performance of jobs as an obligation to serving citizens.

Vaccines today are an exclusive class of drugs given exceptional privileges since 1986. Other pandemics and outbreaks have warranted concern and a sudden push for vaccine advocacy, but COVID-19 is elevating the concern to a different level. Many authorities and scientists quickly point to the Spanish flu outbreak in 1918, which was profoundly serious, but would be more manageable with antibiotics available today. In fact, COVID would be more manageable with proper resources and access to proper antibiotics, antivirals, and other biologic resources available today. The flaws in preparation falls to our government and medical professionals which have failed on many occasions to address and prepare for infectious outbreaks, most notably being authorities and medical professionals granted discretion to make medical and healthcare professional judgement calls for our citizens.

I will briefly cover the Black Plague later which for some odd reason is mentioned in the discussions of our current outbreaks as in some fashion being related to pandemics, but COVID-19 and the Black Plague are far from being related. The Black Plague was an infectious outbreak that involved a bacterial infection, caused by the bacteria *y. pestis* and potentially other bacteria and viruses concurrently or in waves across many societies during the Middle Ages (centuries ago). The Black Plague was a major series of infectious outbreaks that changed many societies for centuries. Today, the Black Plague is often unfairly tied to many infectious disease outbreaks. The Black Plague today is preventable and treatable, not by vaccines, but by antibiotics and good healthcare and sanitary practices. Many individuals forget their history, drug history lessons, and suggest a plague is a part of the widespread cycle of the current infectious outbreaks, which it is not. The science and historical lessons learned are similar for many infectious outbreaks, but many citizens lack understanding that the concerns are not the same, as science, medicine and technology have changed and improved dramatically since the Middle Ages.

A modern concern found today is the threat of bacteria and viruses being used as biological weapons. Spread by novel methods, but if any nation began such a war, who could stop it? Probably no one nation has all the resources and tools needed to stop a biological war where infectious pathogens are used as weapons. Such a war would not be an end of the world type of scenario, but certainly would be an economic game changer, and a threat to destabilizing humanity. All countries ban the use of biological weapons. Such biological weapons still exist, and all nations of earth must work together to address inappropriate use and harm that could be caused by such weapons to many societies. One tool often considered as a neutralizing pharmaceutical tool for biological weapons are vaccines. Unfortunately, there is not a vaccine ready and available for all potentially deadly biological pathogens released as weapons, as such novel vaccines are currently unsafe and ineffective, often stuck in a lab awaiting solutions to adverse complications. The lack of medical tools and resources is a global concern, and perhaps all nations should band together to address all drug concerns for treating such infectious diseases and noted as being related to safety concerns. Vaccine and drug safety are not uniformly addressed through partnerships among nations today. Each country currently operates independently in how they address, evaluate, approve and report ADRs for all drugs, and more specifically all vaccines.

Even where we have checks and balances mechanisms for addressing claims made in science and law, there remains many failures and flawed legal decisions which must also be corrected, and it is our citizens' duty to ensure these errors in science and legal practices are corrected. Government authorities will not correct flawed laws and understandings unless required to do so by citizens. Citizens must be fair and knowledgeable of all drug concerns that affect all citizens. And when necessary, citizens must jump ahead of authorities, if that is what it takes, as many authorities have clearly shown they will make little effort to be informed themselves. A powerful citizen-driven checks and balances battle often must correct flawed and false actions made by authorities in our government on a regular basis.

Flawed vaccine concerns require a broad discussion of science, history, politics, and law. A much broader discussion than this book allows, and certainly with more experts than I bring to this book. In many cases, I do not call the government's experts, "experts", as I find our government's experts make statements that are full of lies, perjury and bias. Government experts, suggested as being the voice of our government, often state one position based on some selected pieces of evidence, but readily change their position or message often for compensation where no referential evidence or facts are presented to support their newfound point-of-view, and then flip again as they feel the need to restate their position again for no apparent justification beyond monetary gain or self-interests. I suggest this is a discretionary action and a flawed act by designated experts of our government, as the experts often have slanted bias and often draw conclusions with limited facts and often even less scientific evidence. What makes an expert change their position? Citizens have a right to know, and it should be based on science and facts, and not changes in personal opinions, or in the case of vaccines, an expert's sudden financial interest and self-interest as a vaccine-involved expert with related interest in vaccine development and promotion. Or in short, financial-driven actions are inappropriate foundations for building public trust as the government's expert is clearly lacking expertise.

I hope to provoke citizens to force our government to make changes. Where there is a need to change or end a foolish vaccine law and affiliated programs that were poorly developed using the Vaccine Act, with perpetually weak administrative oversight. Individual rights should not be unlawfully taken from citizens, as these are basic rights we cherish as a democratic nation. We cannot simply ignore adverse drug risks and concerns and hope for better future outcomes, as this is also the type of wishful thinking that leads to future troubling setbacks. It is inappropriate for any authority to suggest vaccines are completely safe and effective, or that such safety can be pulled out of a hat when there is little data to base such claims on, and what will the results be if such novel and rapidly-developed vaccines actually cause injuries to citizens. There is no flexible and discretionary science for vaccine safety, only discretionary laws to allow compensation at the discretion of a single judge in the Vaccine Injury Compensation Program (also known as the VICP) known as special masters. The special masters are not specialists in science or medicine, but manipulative legal practitioners in law.

Our government plays irresponsibly with science and medical facts. And not just a few authorities and experts acting on behalf of our government, but many parties who collectively act as the voice of our government. Many citizens may not understand, as we are regularly lied to, but a single authority acting as the voice of our government in any government matter, is in fact the voice of our government. And when they lie and cause harm, it is a harm to all citizens and our government. And our government does not have to take action to correct such harms, in fact such harms are often ignored and not addressed. These acts of silence and ignorance are simple acts of political and judicial rudeness, and such acts happen too often in our society.

Sometimes we must step back and look at the facts. As the authorities are not correct, but often are purely guessing for the sake of being speedy, swift, and forming a biased narrative in some fashion. Authorities are also curt and gruff, because they do not like to be questioned on their opinions. Government authorities are like a home team in a sporting event; they often have all the advantages to come home with a win. Individuals are the underdogs, and often carry the burden of being required to be superior in facts and strategy. Americans often cheer for the underdogs, not just because they are the individuals, but because we cheer for facts that make us a better society. The scientific proofs relating to science must be presented and available for all to understand. A little magic is good in science, but in the end, science requires verifiable proofs and facts. Superior facts and evidence proven in science always wins. I personally push for science that is understood, or at least well-founded, and is documented in widely recognized literature. Our government pushes for anything that supports their financial and promotional policies. I professionally reference experts in the field of vaccines and immunology, like Dr. Albert Sabin, Dr. Jonas Salk, Dr. Joseph Bellanti to name a few great American experts in the medical field. These experts looked to address vital and important vaccine questions and concerns.

Transparency and open-minded discussions lead to equality, discoveries, and justice for all. Our government authorities do not offer transparency, and certainly are not receptive to open-minded discussions, but offer more of an authoritative beat down, which is presented with unreliable authoritative bias that citizens are supposed to accept without question. I for one refuse to accept such nonsense. For authorities often wave the flag of science but do not give any scientific documents or literature to support their claims. This is a common and ongoing concern these days and will likely continue to injure many citizens if the current vaccine law and vaccine programs are not addressed by citizens.

For a different perspective on the vaccine market, rather than just thinking of drugs, think of a novel automobile being developed, promoted, pre-ordered from a manufacturer(s) at a profit to be distributed to its citizens and citizens around the world. If there are defects, well the government will pay for any injuries and damages, but you will need to prove the cause of those injuries to a single judge appointed by the government, who individually helped develop the whole legal arrangement and may be a little biased relating to injury compensation, which the government gladly stated they will readily cover to all parties with noted injuries related to the operation of the vehicle. Does this sound like a sweet deal for the automotive manufacturer or shady deal for the consumers? Governments rarely wrap their legal and financial interests this deeply around single commercial products. In fact, it is fundamentally not allowed per constitutional law, but no worries, as citizens are both the receiver of the implied benefits of the vaccine, and citizens (our government) are the safety net, should that undetermined defect ever develop. Vaccines are a special, protected class of drugs indeed.

I will dig a little deeper into vaccine issues in this book covering the National Childhood Vaccine Injury Act of 1986, the Vaccine Information Statements provided by the Centers for Disease Control and Prevention (the CDC), the Vaccine Injury Compensation Program (VICP) administered by the Department of Justice and federal courts, the Vaccine Adverse Effects from Vaccine Reaction (VAERS) reporting programs, and many other parts of our government policies intertwined with our vaccine manufacturers and other vaccine related programs. A mammoth government presence and their understood interest in the success of vaccines. Even though such broad support is not fully championed by all scientists as being essential or required in addressing public health concerns.

As you will learn, I did not wake up one day and say you know what, I need to write a book on vaccines, vaccine safety and our government's vaccine programs. I have my reasons, and they are both personal and professional. Everyone should learn more about vaccines, even the doctors who missed a few classes in medical school on the subject. And all citizens and medical professionals need to learn more about the Vaccine Act and our vaccine programs and suggestive vaccine promotional programs. You will discover vaccine ignorance is not bliss, unless of course bliss is ignorance.

Our healthcare system is failing in many ways. Corruption and self-interest actions run deep in our government, at every level and in every branch of our government. Can we fix these noted conflicts of interest? I do not believe we can fix them in a day, or even a year. Our actions must be firm and long-term, as we must demand safety in our drugs, all drugs; and facts of injury for all drugs, including vaccines. Is it political? Not really, as all government parties have an interest in vaccines succeeding, both financially and for public health concerns. But vaccines are often used as political tools to manipulate the citizens demanding some action which may or may not entirely be for good health.

This book is not a pro-vaccine versus anti-vaccine argument but is a prochoice argument for the express interest of individuals being informed with facts and given informed consent choices. Citizens must always be allowed to make an informed drug decision, also known in medical circles as informed consent before taking any drug or undergoing any medical procedure. The choice can be made with nominal medical information and such choices are made every day where citizens forego their rights and permit a doctor to make a medical judgement in their professional medical opinion as to how to treat a specific medical condition or concern using drugs or medical procedures to correct the suspected medical disorder. It is always the individual's choice to be informed and demand or ask for more information and be allowed to make the right fully informed decision. It is also the doctor and pharmacist's legal duty to supply a medical check and balance professional judgement call if you care to ask for assistance in making an informed consent decision. Many patients do not ask for first or second opinions, but simply accept the first offer of a professional medical opinion, and decline further discussions or understanding, which I will state is often a bad idea.

Most doctors understand the science of vaccines well, especially from a clinical standpoint. Go for deeper pharmacological actions, and you may want a pharmacist investigating all drug concerns and adverse risks. And to go even deeper on such concerns, you probably need a medical researcher, often found in the global marketplace. Vaccine science is both simple and complex. Doctors and the public often understand the simple protective mechanisms of developing immunity to an infectious disease. But for an understanding of vaccine causational mechanisms and pharmaceutical actions, pharmacists, vaccine researchers, and medical researchers contribute greater understanding of vaccine science. Government authorities prefer to stick with the simple and easy message for citizens to easily comprehend, like vaccines are protective and "generally" safe, and not that vaccines may cause serious adverse events which can be difficult to manage and treat.

Our government states, using its broad interpretative legal advantages authorized by the Vaccine Act, that citizens do not need to understand causational mechanisms to understand and file claims of vaccine injuries, but I would advise citizens differently. A citizen must be exceptionally well educated in vaccines and their actions to argue a vaccine injury. And if a citizen is unconcerned with the possibility of an adverse vaccine injury, the citizen may be walking a tight-rope with no safety net, where the tight-rope may be two feet off the ground or 2000 feet off the ground. Citizens must listen to scientists who make observations and test mechanisms of drug actions and understand the science. Understanding the application of the discretional Vaccine Law and vaccine science is mandatory and is not optional. Opinions and beliefs of the VICP administrative judges often make no sense, even where medical professionals and citizens point to science that has been observed and is mostly understood through scientific research.

I am not in favor of demanding any citizen take any particular action regarding any drug, but simply encourage citizens must become informed citizens, and can learn lessons and knowledge from my many years of knowledge gained through pharmacy practices and focused probing into vaccine research. Vaccines are not my life or livelihood, but have dramatically impacted my life, and even more dramatically impacted my child's life. I have experienced the inept medical and legal professionals who lay claim to being our government's experts in vaccines and addressing vaccine safety concerns through the VICP program and other federal agencies. My interests are concerns for all citizens, and the flawed path our government offers for supplying and addressing vaccine safety. I hope you enjoy the book, and I hope you choose to become active in choices you can make which will impact vaccine safety for all citizens.

CHAPTER 1

Ushering in Vaccine Inc.

As a point of introduction, I will say up front I have always found vaccines to be a challenging subject to introduce. Should the lesson start with how vaccines work? Or should the message start with which vaccines an individual needs and when they need them? Do we start with the history, or the science? And do discussions talk about the scientists and their discoveries, and what vaccine facts they have learned over time? Or do we simply glaze over the science, and suggest why we need to vaccinate in accordance with CDC guidelines, as the CDC prefers, we consider all vaccines vital? Introduction to vaccines are a strange starting point of conversation. Every person has a typical set of lessons they learned in school, if they learned anything at all about vaccines and what vaccines do. It is kind of like talking about sex. Some teachers give you the 30-second brief over lesson on vaccines and immunity, and some children and adults were taught about vaccines from information they likely learned on the playground. If there is a national standard lesson on vaccines in schools, I have not seen the lessons beyond how vaccines cause the immune system to develop antibodies and protective immunity. There are textbooks on immunology and vaccines, and the CDC and other resources offer websites and information on how vaccines work. These lessons are limited in scope, often with inadequate discussion of mechanisms of action and adverse events linked to vaccines. Injuries from adverse drug reactions relating to vaccines are an advanced topic that few parties care to learn about or address even in a professional setting.

As much as I like vaccines as a subject matter and I truly like the author of some of the best textbooks on the subject of immunology, I will not be digging too deeply into the science here, as I believe most readers will simply stop reading my book. The mechanisms of how vaccines act on the immune system to help develop antibodies is largely an understood mechanism of action inside the body's immune system. The observed actions of vaccine processes and immunologic system responses are higher-level science discovered in the last few decades. Not necessarily the top discoveries in science, but vaccines are highly significant immunologic discoveries. When the patient receives a vaccine, the vaccine contains distinctive particulate matter called antigens that activate the cells of the immune system, and the patient then develops antibodies that help form the protection in their body against future infections primarily from the same infectious disease as the antigens originated. The CDC's website gives a basic explanation of how vaccines work, noted at: www.cdc.gov/vaccines/hcp/conversations/downloads/vacsafe-understand-color-office.pdf (or simply type in: Understanding How Vaccines Work in a search engine), which provides a novice explanation for beginners and those refamiliarizing themselves with how vaccines work. The CDC website is also steadfastly managed to relay a promotional message for the government agencies and physician associations that support, prescribe, and administer vaccines to many adults and children through most primary care healthcare practices, noted on several CDC documents as a message which is advocated in conjunction with the American Academy of Family Physicians and the American Academy of Pediatrics physicians.

While I understand the physicians' advocacy support for vaccines, many doctors generally miss the boat on adverse vaccine injuries. The support for vaccine efficacy (also called effectiveness) has always been strongly supported by medical professionals, but vaccine injuries and adverse events are often left to be discussed as secondary concerns. I appreciate the implied need for vaccines as I have read through numerous vaccine guidelines and professional literature on vaccines over the last five decades, but case reports and medical literature on adverse vaccine reactions have not been covered as well, when compared to other classes of drugs. Most healthcare parties simply call vaccines protective medicine, as vaccines are not used to treat a disease but help the body develop antibodies for protection. An inactivated antigen acts as an "innocent" foreign agent introduced into the body which many professionals suggest causes no "real" harm to the body. Some even suggesting, an adverse reaction is in general a good thing. This book will cover some of these not so innocent adverse vaccine injuries, along with the government's vaccine programs, vaccine law and broad general statements our government's authorities often make about vaccines. I will try to focus on the current state of vaccines, and not the law or science, as I will give you access to extended details on those for free online, if you care to learn more details about a vaccine injury case the government "secretly" manages.

To fill the gaps left by physicians, I have chosen to begin this book with a look at how normal citizens view vaccines today. A sort of word association, I say vaccines and you, the reader, would say? Protection. Family. Stop Infections. Employment. You know the word vaccine, what does it mean to the citizens? Let us start there. That is what the

CDC, WHO, and other vaccine advocacy groups recommend that I start with, when I am told to advise patients professionally about vaccines from a benefits only perspective.

I am told, “do not start with the science”, but focus on the protection provided by vaccines, which can be a bit misleading. We are told you will lose the attention of a patient in less than 30 seconds if you start with the science. Start with the things that matter to the patient, like family. You want to protect your family and yourself. You want to protect your community and society in general. All good talking points for an advertisement. And what you may often find on a poster for vaccines.

This does not mean patients do not want to understand the science, as I can usually spot the scientists in the group at the beginning of a discussion. Often, they have already made up their mind and know what they want, as the science is somewhat understood, so we can often just skip the explanation and go straight to the shot. Occasionally, I must explain how the vaccine will be administered, and what to expect as a possible adverse side effect, and of course provide a Vaccine Information Statement (also called a VIS) from the CDC. For many vaccines, the VIS provides a common list of adverse vaccine reactions, but the list is noticeably short, and covers only the few common side effects which occur in over 10% of the patients vaccinated. The Vaccine Information Statement which is required to be provided by the vaccinating health care provider prior to a vaccination has often been known to get lost in the stacks of paper and coupons you may get at the pharmacy, or healthcare professionals forget how to print the VIS if they cannot find it nearby when they are ready to administer the vaccine.

You should always receive a VIS as a bare minimum of information when you agree to be vaccinated. Just request the doctor, or pharmacist provide you with the VIS if you are not given one at the time of vaccination. I also recommend a current professional full prescribing disclosure statement (also called professional package inserts, or simply a PI statement) as approved by the FDA and created as a professional reference by the vaccine manufacturer for medical professionals to read through and learn possible risks and warnings related to the vaccine being administered. The PI statements are sometimes in a consumer and professional version, I would ask for the professional version and request explanation of medical jargon as needed. Most medical jargon definitions are available online, but any medical professional can also assist in understanding the terminology.

Medical professionals often discuss vaccine details and mechanisms with patients but many of the discussions are short and incomplete. Perhaps a brief discussion on how vaccines are injected into the body and your body responds to the antigens, occasionally explaining how a deactivated (generally not live, but some are live and inactivated viruses) viral strain are designed to trigger an immune response when it is injected into your muscle tissue and subsequently circulates through the blood to your immune system to create antibodies in your body to help you fight off future viral infections linked to a corresponding pathogen. The process of developing antibodies takes a few weeks to months, so even as patients proudly show others their stylish vaccination promotional sticker saying that they were recently jabbed, the inoculated person will not develop immunity from the vaccine for several weeks or longer following the jab. Some doctors like to inform the patient the protection will start faster stating "some protection early is better than no protection", but this is mostly a positive reinforcing promotional statement, as protection does not kick in immediately and generally depends on your body's immune cell responses. The general idea of getting protected from an infectious disease with a single shot however is a powerful image to most citizens who simply want to avoid getting sick from the infectious pathogens covered by a particular vaccine.

Many patients mistakenly proclaim protection from infections start shortly after being vaccinated, but the process is much more complex and not as simple as just getting a vaccine shot. The process of developing immunity again takes weeks. However, the process of provoking an adverse body system response to the vaccine can happen quickly, some positive and expected responses, and sometimes negative adverse reactions occurring in seconds to hours after the shot, and sometimes the responses occur over months after the injection. Body system responses are not the same as immune system protective mechanism responses understood to lead to the development of antibodies. The process of provoking an immune system response takes days, before specialized immune cells known as T-cells and B-cells begin to act and stimulate the development of antibodies. In between this time, the vaccine is still circulating around the body and causing other body system events, from localized inflammation to other actions on various cell tissue. Your body reacts to these adverse reactionary events, as it would with any other injection of a foreign substance. Some are responses known as atopy or allergic responses and others are tied to a general response, like inflammation, to a foreign substance being injected into your body, which various organs and systems begin a process of trying to eliminate, by responding to the foreign substance, isolating the foreign substance, and finding routes to eliminate the foreignness, which is considered a normal body mechanical response process.

The process is not universally the same for all patients, and sometimes the response can be serious or complicating to a patient with underlying medical conditions or for patients at different ages. Or serious and complicating to patients that were previously viewed as perfectly normal and healthy individuals prior to the vaccine injection. The general idea and hope are that these responses are temporary and will go away through a process of healing and repair, commonly called a return to homeostasis (or balance), which means a patient's body will find balance again, just as it does when you get sick and recover for an infectious illness. The same process, but hopefully shorter and less problematic, is the general hope.

But what if the balancing process is more complicated than expected? What will happen next? That is an area of a lot of uncertainty and speculative medicine, and not just speculations by average doctors, but also from specialists which may need to address the adverse events often starting in an emergency room. The doctors may treat it as a typical infection-like response, with prescribed drugs for symptoms and prescribed rest for a typical onset of complications often related to being like having the illness. Rarely, the medical events may lead to broad inflammation, and a need for antibiotics to treat a bacterial infection , not a new bacterium, but often bacteria your body already has present either inside your body or on your skin. These types of adverse complications are not considered common, but are entirely possible, as your body often triggers a response far beyond the simple immune responses the doctors explain as common side effects when they are administering the vaccine. It is a normal biological process often driven by a mechanical process called mimicry which mimics a body's normal infectious disease response. Doctors often expect the lesser noted complications to fade away, but sometimes the body does not respond as expected.

The more serious complications that can occur are the adverse reactions found inside the body's cell tissues, circulating proteins found in the blood, and interacting directly with organ tissue. Impacting various biological systems and perhaps changing how these organs and body systems work. Among scientists, it is often called cell-to-cell communication, as cells change and communicate with other cells to tell each cell what they should do under differing response scenarios. Not every cell in your body jumps into action, but over time every cell is likely exposed to some type of cellular response mechanisms. These are again thought to be normal responses, but what you see on the outside of the patient's body is not the whole picture and may differ from what is going on inside the body.

I say this, as this is a simplified explanation of how drugs in general work inside your body. Drugs that are taken orally, inhaled, applied to the skin and through other routes of administration often behave a little differently from drugs that are injected directly into your body intramuscularly or directly into the blood. The desired targeted action of the drug is generally the same by any route of administration, which is to treat a specific ailment, but the body's responses often differ based on several factors. Most vaccines are no different from other drugs in this respect as the method of delivery does not make the vaccine any safer or less likely to cause a drug injury. But the sequence and triggers of circulating cells is often quite different, as injected vaccines cause cell mechanism changes in several organs, including the spleen, liver, and other vital organs.

Any implied safety promoted by medical professionals when administering a vaccine injection is purely a psychological calming suggestion (what your mind thinks), as the drug will certainly cause a physiological response (what your body seeks to accomplish) once injected. What that response will be is not always certain, and doctors will generally not speculate until they judge it as necessary to make an appropriate diagnosis and begin treatment for the adverse event, which may not occur immediately, but can occur over several hours or several days later after the vaccination injection. When and how an impacted patient is treated is largely based on clinical data and professional judgement calls made by a treating physician who will evaluate selective clinical findings. If the treating physician has seen the problem before, the adverse events may be addressed quickly. If the adverse response is new to the doctor, it may be addressed more slowly or may be missed entirely as an adverse event. In which case, the complication could become much worse or your body may go through a response mechanism and again find balance through homeostatic processes. The natural process of finding balance is the most favored progression doctors expect your body to do to return back to good health. A less favorable process of developing other medical complications which can be complex and involve multiple body systems can be difficult to assess and treat, and sometimes leads to medical complications that are difficult to manage.

Medical professionals are not perfect, and the drug science is complicated. So, it is understandable the doctors will rarely uncover the serious vaccine-related complications and suggest the chance of an injury relating to a vaccine as suggestively being a rare occurrence. That does not mean vaccine injuries do not happen, but the injuries are less frequently documented, and are less common than the 10% or greater group of adverse side effects often discussed with patients prior to injection, as many serious adverse events occur in the less than a 1% range rate of occurrence. But when serious adverse reactions do occur, most medical professional do not have the training or resources to handle many complicated adverse vaccine reactions. Doctors generally refer such cases to the emergency room for immediate attention and will often request clinical tests which may show where the complications are occurring in the body. Perhaps a dysfunctional organ or genetic-specific issues that was not known prior to the vaccine injection which was not expected, or perhaps the vaccine complication is age related or medical condition related, where the doctors may offset the argument with "the adverse event could have happened anyway, regardless of the vaccine". In other words, you might be a ticking timebomb just waiting to go off no matter what, the vaccine could have been involved in initiating the complication, but the doctors do not know for sure. Some will often state the vaccine probably had nothing to do with the adverse vaccine reaction, which is generally an insincere statement to deflect the discussion of what may have originated as a vaccine-related injury. This is not magic or undiscovered science, but this is science and a pharmacological response vaccine injury mechanism, often called a vaccine-induced adverse biological response to a vaccination.

A patient having a serious adverse event will often be directed to a hospital emergency room where doctors order basic health data information and blood samples from the patient to address immediate treatment actions to stabilize the patient's health. Emergency room doctors will rarely, if ever, look at a vaccine adverse reaction as a primary cause of injury unless it is obviously related in some manner to something they have learned or a doctor has seen as a vaccine-related complication in their medical experiences. Doctors often immediately look to the patient's medical history, as doctors will likely point to some previous medical condition perhaps triggering a medical crisis. Or if not there, a family history of a medical condition, or other medications, or illicit drugs the patient may have taken. Anything but the vaccine, as vaccine injuries are way down the list of injuries doctors look for answers to bring the body's systems back into balance. In general, normal blood work will lead them to prescribe rest and observation, and standard symptomatic treatment plans, and mark the event as an irregular reaction which they often mark as idiopathic (or they do not know the cause for what happened). The number of adverse event cases labelled as idiopathic represents over 50% of all reported cases of hospitalization and death in statistical reporting.

I state the importance of these more complex medical complications as scientists and medical professionals often look for simple answers and simple treatment plans, without a complete evaluation of possible vaccine-induced medical complications. The complex problems are often left to specialist to address if there is a knowledgeable specialist available to address the concern. Otherwise everyday practitioners will look for issues and try to figure them out based on data and information provided by lab reports, and statements by federal agencies like the FDA, who in turn rely on manufacturers to provide up-to-date data and information, which is often not up-to-date but often 10 to 15 years old.

It takes years, and often decades, for the FDA to evaluate and decide the proper inclusion of some adverse drug events in drug literature, which were not included in the initial application for approval of a drug, requiring further evaluation as to the need to be added as a newer adverse risk. The understanding that reliable medical information is available through dependable medical resources is not consistently true today. Many doctors do not use up-to-date reliable resources considered current within the last few decades, as some professionals use medical literature resources which would now be considered out-of-date. In today's world, technology makes a lot of current resources available, but many medical professionals simply have no time to stay up to date without being incentivized or mandated.

Can important and vital drug data and drug complications be ignored or overlooked as they relate to adverse events? Yes, and it happens a lot. As I mentioned, the FDA commissioner and other regulatory agencies are given wide discretion to allow drugs and prescribing practices to operate under a broad umbrella of practice methods and knowledge collectively called "good faith" efforts by all parties understood to be practicing inside the public and patient's best interest. This is not a fact-based process of addressing medicine and medical concerns, but regulatory agencies operate under a discretionary-based administrative practices, often driven by fees and penalties which are paid to the agency and support salaries and staffing. This occurs at both the federal and state levels.

At the FDA, manufacturers are given discretion to address concerns in a slow systematic process which also benefits the manufacturer who simply wants to make a profit and recoup and replenish costs for research and development. Where pharmaceutical profits can be enormous, but there is only limited interest in researching and addressing rare adverse medical concerns. And even when such medical concerns are reported as an adverse event, proper regulatory actions are often slowed by bureaucratic practices of stalling or even the occasional monetary conflicts of interests among interconnected parties.

Our drug laws at both the federal and state levels provide broad discretionary powers granted to multiple agency leaders, which oddly conflict with mandated actions formally required in drug laws. Drug laws state the agency leaders must address drug injuries and adverse events relating to any drug with no regard or discretion given to "any particulars", which specifically means the drug-related agencies must address all safety concerns in an immediate fashion once the adverse concern is made known to the agency. This rule would imply public safety and addressing drug safety is a highly-important primary concern to all agencies but does not properly address the flip side of drug laws which gives administrative and legal professionals in the agency broad discretionary powers to do nothing, or push a problem down the road, often getting lost in turnover of staff or the commissioners themselves. Or complaints and concerns are untraceably passed to a "team of experts" who often fail in performing their assigned job duties to address the noted concerns. It is often a bureaucratic cycle of wasted red tape. But who is looking at such waste? Government auditors and oversight committees with an eye on efficiency, and not failed job performance.

And if the agencies are a flawed or incompetent agency, who cares other than a few legislators interested in playing a political game with hopes of lowering an agency's funding, as few legislated programs rarely go completely away in our government. Vaccine programs are inexplicably wrapped around multiple agencies often duplicating job functions. Many drug-related agencies have a poor performance track record as noted by way of internal auditors. Who pays for these failed drug agencies? The public pays for our government's inefficiencies and failures. The agencies often assign failures to being underfunded or understaffed as reasons for not addressing many concerns in a timely manner for the public or medical professionals, which is both sad, and as they would say, unfortunate. For example, the staff of the FDA will often say something like, "The FDA staff was not made aware of an adverse drug reaction discovered 20 years ago and did not get around to properly addressing the risk until recently, and it took the FDA staff another 10 years to review it and issue a warning. And it is just unfortunate your loved one was harmed or died. All drugs have uncertain risks". This is not a joke about the FDA and many federal agencies, but this is a reality-based approach to drug regulation and addressing drug concerns, and especially vaccine safety issues. In a better world, if a government agency is incapable of doing its job efficiently, then the agency would logically need to be eliminated, or at least revamped. Collectively today, we have way too much government fat and overlapping duties at all levels of government. Drug regulation and vaccine-related parties today are an entirely useless collection of agencies, which collectively do not address drug safety or public safety.

Multiple agencies, even overlapping agencies in the same governmental departments often provide conflicting and inaccurate information, which are simply unforgivable excuses. I mention these drug concerns as we have a current elevated infectious outbreak where drug errors and misstatements can be critical to citizen and public health. As such errors can lead to bias and promotion of a cause for actions which are not transparently justified, where adverse risks are minimalized using authoritative discretions to rush approvals based on good faith efforts, which falsely suggests proficiency in addressing an imminent threat.

The current pandemic known as COVID-19 was found, reported, and first addressed in China in late 2019. The originating source is currently unknown, and many of its characteristics are also uncertain, as it is a novel virus. The virus is highly contagious and has been suggested as being a contagion, a serious pandemic; but the current threat-level is not at the level of being a contagion. Many patients infected are not seriously affected or function as normal citizens completely absent of any symptoms, also referred to as being asymptomatic. Widespread speculation has caused a media and medical profession mania, which is somewhat justified given the lack of information and historical lag in government reporting. Testing, treatment protocols, and other medical protocols are all lagging, as this is a novel virus. Many officials act as if there was never a plan to address such an infectious outbreak regardless of the novel nature of the infection. For the record, most hospitals and public health agencies make at least some attempt at training for an emergency infectious outbreak, but few are prepared for anything more than a seasonal spike-type infectious disease outbreak. Some doctors and public health leaders panic in a mild flu outbreak.

Where did cool, calm and collected professionals go? Maybe those classes were cut, both here and abroad, from the medical curriculum for classes needed to graduate.

Government authorities attempt to address public health concerns with fast moving data and sometimes use wild analytical and statistical models. Not that they have not done this before in past infectious disease outbreaks. To complicate matters, authorities also spread fear of multiple infectious diseases, which will only heighten the numbers of medical complications, and of course deaths. These are not facts being disputed here but are speculative explanations of how our government works and often misuses data and science to send a flawed message to its citizens which demands submission to authorities rather than a calm and rational discussion of concerns and steady application of scientific actions.

Theoretical science has always been exactly that, hypothetical, using many assumed facts when facts are uncertain. All facts related to COVID-19 and other novel infections are mostly speculative, and not fully known at this early stage of learning details related to the virus circulating in several populations. In fact, many statements are nonspecific infectious disease statements and are assigned as being PIC infections, which are Pneumonia (bacterial)-Influenza (viral)-and/or Coronaviruses (viral). When testing for any of these infectious diseases, if a positive COVID-19 test result is discovered COVID is generally labelled as the primary source of any further medical complications. Multiple infections and medical complications relating to a preexisting condition could be very problematic. Testing is not perfect, and epidemiologists and statisticians simply fill in the gaps until more useful testing data is developed. Statisticians and other medical records theorists are often not physicians but are assigned as collectors of data and reporting records to designate certain infections as primary sources of injury and complications, including death. COVID-19 is the most frequently listed primary infectious "disease of the day" for reporting purposes. Currently, if a patient has a positive COVID test, all other medical and infectious concerns are shifted to being listed as secondary. So COVID data can skewer all other medical statistical data in order of suggested importance by medical professionals with only limited medical training.

I state this fact not to dismiss concerns for public health but to point out that many statements regarding public health are speculative and uncertain. The public should know this fact and be concerned with statistics until a significant scientific conclusion can be drawn from facts and fully understood, which does not fit the media model for facts which are often released as fast as possible in line with the public's desire for immediate news. Disappointingly, doctors and medical professionals fall into the same trap, but such convoluted facts are nothing new. These types of fact-bending statements and misstatements have gone on for centuries. Why stop now when the public simply wants to be satisfied immediately by speculative facts in a social media-style immediate release of instant news? Sensationalist yellow journalism has a history that parallels the history of vaccines. Drama and sensational headlines are designed to sell advertising and is often used to impact politics and public opinion. Nothing new here, public consumption of poorly prepared science has been going on for centuries.

Government agencies try to satisfy the people by pushing vaccines as an answer to an infectious disease, especially emphasizing vaccine effectiveness and inexplicably disregarding vaccine safety concerns. The prerequisite risk-to-benefit analysis of vaccines is slanted not for the citizens to understand safety concerns but to aid medical professionals in promoting vaccines to the masses. Do car salespeople sell defective cars? Sure, they do, that is what recalls are for, and warranty servicing. Vaccine "sales professionals" do not intentionally sell defective products, but it happens and hopefully nothing bad comes as a result of the vaccine misunderstood defect. Currently, our government authorities proclaim, "they will protect us", but the human body is far more complicated to address from a mechanical perspective compared to a car. Vaccine-related injuries are not just a maybe-type of concern but are a highly likely adverse event that could be just around the corner. Many vaccine-related injuries are unfortunately shamefully swept under the government's rug of shame.

In short, the human body has many discovered adverse vaccine reactions, but the public seems unaware vaccine drug facts are NOT considered under the same rules and requirements for drug safety standards as all drugs. Vaccines fall into an exclusive and elusive class of drugs. Vaccine drug-class legal protections are mostly a result of a law enacted in 1986 called the *National Childhood Vaccine Injury Act* (also referred to as the Vaccine Act or Vaccine Law). Not that it had much to do with children, but it was a good selling point to get the Law passed, signed, and enacted. In fact, over 30 years later, many parties in our government still think it is primarily for children, but the law covers all patients injured by vaccines regardless of their age.

To this day, most doctors and medical professionals have only a limited idea of what the Vaccine Law is and do not know much beyond there is a law that was mentioned somewhere (not on the board exams needed to get licensed) but that there is a law that states "some sort of" federal program is supposed to cover an injury relating to a vaccine. In other words, vaccine injuries are covered. Not just serious injuries but all medical and drug liabilities are covered. Just do not ask medical professionals about the details, as that is legal stuff, and doctors hate legal stuff, especially if their practices are excused from the legal concern. Most medical professionals do not know the Vaccine Law is supposed to cover all injury caused by a vaccine, or any injury related to the vaccine which led to further medical complications including an unmanageable preexisting medical condition which becomes further complicated by the vaccine-noted injury.

If this sounds like a complicated medical causational diagnosis, it is, but that is how the government enacted the law listing the vaccine injury coverage requirements in the Vaccine Act. Doctors often have no idea how the law works but politely state the government will cover a vaccine injury without understanding how or what the details of reporting are regarding coverage. And lawyers are equally poorly trained, as most lawyers have no idea what the details of the vaccine law are, but many suggest it is supposed to be a good program. Presumably, they heard it was a good program somewhere by someone.

Both sets of professionals failing to understand the practice of addressing vaccine injuries has shifted to being speculative and whimsical at the discretion of a single government judge called a special master. The special master is a specialized administrative judge who evaluates vaccine injuries, not specifically required to use anything related to vaccine science and medicine. This is not to say they cannot be fair if given the facts, but the vaccine facts are not addressed and presented as facts and evidence which would be addressed under normal constitutional restrictions and court rules as many citizens would recognize as facts and evidence a normal jury would be presented in a normal civil or criminal trial.

Vaccine facts and injury facts are condensed, with numerous limits placed on the number of experts and evidence allowed to be evaluated by the special master. The special master is authorized by the Vaccine Act to use wide discretion to address facts and science relating to how the experts are given brief time to give testimony to present timing and causational relationship of a vaccine injury. Which includes testimony where medical experts are constantly asked to lower their scientific discussions to avoid going over the special master's head, as most special masters have trouble understanding the vaccine-injury science. Simple medical statements and graphics are good but nothing above a grade school level is advised, as the special master might get lost in the vaccine science discussion. To be clear, the Vaccine Injury Compensation Program was established as a program under the Vaccine Act that promised it would favor the injured party and would give substantial weight to the patient's treating physician acting as one of the allowed experts for the party claiming an injury. This promise to doctors and injured patients is often lost in the special master's biased legal discretion and interest in protecting vaccines. Doctors serving as the government's biased vaccine experts make silly and stupid counterarguments to a vaccine-injury claim both before and during a trial, which the special master can allow, or consider okay for a doctor to change their statements "on a whim", as the special master can also change their opinions on an injury claim "in a wink".

The science and medical facts used by special masters are often incorrect facts, and result in misstated facts and misunderstood science used to shape false narratives. One could say to prop-up a mostly false system of promised justice, but that would be too simple. Lawyers created the law. Lawyers reshaped the injury program after getting it enacted. And lawyers certainly gain financially from the law. The primary benefactor of the Vaccine Act however has always been the vaccine/pharmaceutical manufacturers, and by extension the politicians and lawyers lobbying for doctors and manufacturers to protect their interests commercially, personally, and professionally.

For the average citizen, I have often heard parties address vaccines as being compared to something that is magical, as something to be enjoyed, but not much unlike the special masters, not always fully understood. A magician does not explain his secrets, and the magic seems to work, so no one should question the process or methods relating to the magic. The magician looks like a genius and all parties are satisfied. Or at least most parties are generally satisfied and carry on their merry way.

However, the shiny endorsements of a vaccine's protective features start to lose their luster when you peel back the layers and find a multitude of adverse biological side effects. Some of these reactions are not so bad some parties would say, and can be observed by the naked eye, or felt and expressed as a feeling, like pain, or swelling. Other adverse events are more complex and involve a shift in immune system activity, which of course leads to an excess or an overflow of responses by other body systems, often tied to the liver (your endocrine system) or the spleen (your immune/lymphatic system) - two vital regulatory centers of the body's immune-metabolic-endocrine network of regulating systems.

Why are these adverse events important? Because they regulate your body's response to many drugs and act to filter your blood relaying the biological message telling your body what it must do next to respond to an adverse reaction? Vaccines are unique drugs, but they are not unbelievably special drugs that are in some fashion harm-free as many reported adverse biological events occur as understood to be related to adverse vaccine reactions. Some adverse reactions are rapid, while others take days or months to develop. These responses evolve into what the FDA and scientists generally research and catalog as being a drug's safety profile, or others refer to as a listing of risks, adverse effects, warnings, and precautions relative to the suggested use and dosage considerations for any drug.

Drug safety profiles are important because they tell us which responses are complicating, and which responses can be managed, and which may lead to further complications that may be serious and harmful to patients. The longer a drug has been on the market, the better, in general, its safety profile is understood. This is a function of several factors, including more pharmacovigilance reporting (fancy word for drug study safety reporting), more data as reported in case reports from individual cases and studies, and more researchers digging into unknown factors that have led to complications not initially observed visually or noted through some expressed and reported emotion. Safety profiles form the basis of determining which drugs are best included in a treatment protocol, and which drugs have too many complicating factors which can lead to perhaps being considered a drug of last resort or not particularly a good drug choice when compared to other drug protocols and treatment plans.

A general medical assumption is often made that all body systems will eventually, perhaps with pharmaceutical assistance, return to normal function after an adverse event; but what if the body's systems are not in harmony to begin with? Well, that is a complication doctors deal with every day. There is no certainty in diagnosing all medical conditions, and complex factors lead to unexpected biological responses. Doctors have a favorite word for this, it is called idiopathic, which means "we do not know what is going on". And let us, the doctors and patient, just play this out and see what is happening and try to control symptoms and biological factors we can control, with drugs and clinical procedures. For many people, this type of problem often falls into a category we state as, "well that biological response is just unfortunate". Surely, the doctors and scientists learn from these types of complications and teach each other so we can fix the problem for others experiencing the same problem in the future? This is true; that is what science is supposed to be about: test, discover, retest, apply what was learned, and find answers through understood logic and principles, and is meant to be shared with other scientists.

For most scientists, this is a scientific method for isolating and identifying medical complications. For some non-scientists it is magic. Magic of course meaning different things to different groups of people. Highly intelligent people often fall for the wizardry of magic. Where the magician thinks a trick is easy and fun, people pay money to see creativity and illusions. Vaccines are not magic, but many treat the vaccines as magical in some fashion. A wonder drug that leads to good health. Many believe vaccines are pure and good and cause little harm. Nothing too bad, but maybe just a little harm. Patients can get over such harm and still enjoy life. I like to image the parallels and where readers can draw references to what vaccines may mean to you and our society. I want vaccines to be familiar and understandable, something everyone can relate to.

I thought about this and I decided a fair reference now is the book many children have read where citizens look for a golden ticket so they can visit and enjoy all the magical wonders of chocolate. How it is made. The behind the scenes "magic" of how chocolate is prepared and then enjoyed. The story of Willy Wonka (or Charlie if you prefer) & the Chocolate Factory. Delicious chocolates for everyone. There are different types of chocolate for different individuals. Some are preferred over others, but almost everyone loves chocolate. You cannot explain the dangers of chocolate to a chocolate lover, can you? There are none, are there?

Of course, chocolates have their dangers, as you could be allergic. Or maybe you have a medical condition or medication you take that reacts to ingredients in the chocolate or added ingredients that have been mixed in. Or maybe your metabolism just does not process all the chocolate well and you end up obese or develop some other tragic medical problem. These are not problems you say, that is the individual's problem, not the chocolate's fault. You cannot take away chocolates, they are too important, to me and to society. In other words, get your hands off the chocolate and move along, no one should stop providing the things we love, and we can control the bad stuff, if we can just learn lessons from a great story. And, if we really try and teach these lessons to individuals that have the problems, then everything will be okay, and we can all just sit back and enjoy.

Or simply learn chocolates are a simple pleasure, meant to be enjoyed in measured quantities. Everyone is unique, and everyone has a different response and level of reaction to chocolates. It is easy to forget, not everyone has the same biological responses and love for chocolate.

This overboard response is how I image the public feels about vaccines. Not that we love them so much, but to many parties, vaccines are vital to humanity and our existence. What makes them vital to our existence in the eyes of many citizens? We have been told they are vital since we were young children. "Be quiet", we are told, "it will only hurt for a little bit, but this will make you all better and you will be protected forever from getting sick from a bad illness ever again". Or at least until the next year when we do it all over again. An experience a child is taught is part of life and good health.

As you get older, maybe you learn some of the science of antibodies, immunoglobulins, T-cells, B-cells, and other immune system processes. The magical biological activities of your immune system. When something goes wrong in your body or in nature, you can hope to find the golden ticket that will help cure everything and make it all better. Maybe this is a weird jump of perspectives from Willy Wonka to vaccines, but lessons must start somewhere. Personally, I like to think of the vaccine world as the Wacky, Wonky World of Vaccine Inc.

Vaccine Inc is a far different world than you know and live in. It is a world most people certainly do not understand or even try to understand. In fact, there is too much to understand and not enough true answers to relate to your everyday life. The Vaccine Incorporated world I know is probably far different from the medical world you know and heard of in the media and from your doctors and other healthcare providers. Certainly, different from the lessons your teachers taught you in school. Vaccine Inc, like Willy Wonka Inc, is an uncontrolled monster of a business, that directly and indirectly links together hundreds of businesses and government agencies under a single shared interest, collectively known to the public as the promotional advocacy of vaccines and vaccinations. A bit dramatic, you say. No not really, but fascinating when you look at the roles the players play in the real world.

Vaccine manufacturers and researchers serve multiple parties. They do not take a collective oath to do no harm, but pledge to search for discoveries and answers to illness. If parties are harmed, hopefully it will be a lab animal, and not a human. But if it is a human, hopefully scientists will catch the injury quickly and can limit the harm. This experimental process is known as clinical lab trials. Where scientists test drugs to see if they truly do what we expect them to do, based upon our earlier experience with drugs similar in structure and mechanism of action.

Citizens often become the vaccine mass-market test subjects while acting as the end user of Vaccine Inc's consumer products. Where clinical trials will hopefully iron out misunderstood science, and a more generally understood safety profile can hopefully be presented to the medical community at large, who in turn will educate the masses of its benefits and adverse risks. As this decision-making process advances citizen's understanding of the need and use for the vaccine, and the citizen makes the ultimate choice, is the vaccine the right drug or medical procedure for you? As vaccine risks and benefits become more clearly defined.

A comparable consumer-business relationship exists for many commercial products, like automobiles. Car companies develop vehicles that fit your needs and function, sometimes in unique and interesting ways. The cars must work as regulated, must be sufficiently interesting to sell, must be serviced when they do not work as advertised, and they must be held liable if they are defective or cause injury in any manner. All normal and expected factors that would help you decide which car you want to buy.

A little sexy promotion, or creative features, does not hurt either, as everyone wants simplicity and to be pleasing to others. Advertising often pushes the limits of what is true, and what is real from a functional standpoint. But what if there were no serious limits in what could be said in the promotions? The promotional imagination can go wild as there are fewer limits to what can be promoted.

Unlike most commercial products, vaccine manufacturers often have this special privilege to explore science and explore promotion. In fact, the government does most of the promotion for vaccine manufacturers, so the manufacturers do not have to get caught in a lie. The government, the masters of spin, will fix the messages and information, to make vaccines look great. Can you imagine the world we would live in if we had the government promoting all our commercial products? Some countries live in that world and it is not perfect.

I believe this would be called big business-government (or maybe socialism), where we look to our government to give us all of our answers, to be our problem solvers, to be "our parents"? Really, do we want this? A society where you are no longer a citizen but simply an end-product user. This of course is not a form of democracy or capitalism, but some alternative form of governance. One that is different from the founding principles used in writing our Constitution.

Big businesses often work with governments to develop products people may or may not need, as our government often works with businesses directing them on how and when to make certain products. Is that the world we live in today? Yes, it is, but is it the world we want to live in today? Where our government strategizes a plan to be a global leader and selectively tries to corner parts of the scientific business world, which often cannot be cornered? The song *Everybody Wants To Rule The World* comes to mind, and a lot of Vaccine Inc players are playing a political game of who will rule the vaccine world. The fact is no one can rule the vaccine world, as few nations work together on vaccines.

Vaccine manufacturers live in this world. You and I do not, at least not intentionally. We live in a world full of wants and needs, and hopefully products filled with good intentions and outcomes. Vaccine manufacturers suggestively fit this need, so we suggestively want their product.

In the United States, the vaccine companies do not run the vaccine industry, the government does. The vaccine manufacturers are a collection of pharmaceutical manufacturers with ongoing or sufficient manufacturing capacity to make vaccines, often not in the United States, but through various manufacturing plants in numerous countries, often given incentives and tax breaks to be in such countries. Are citizens' interests considered when such decisions are made? Not really. The key factors considered are cost, efficiency and of course profit. This is a foundational basis for any pharmaceutical manufacturer being in the vaccine business.

Sounds like a good business to be in, right? Well it is and it is not for several reasons. Mostly a supply and demand thing, and of course the occasional bad public relations concerns that inevitably comes with the tasks of developing a vaccine. Vaccine manufacturers are generally a different breed of drug manufacturers. Some are dedicated to novel science, like solving an algorithm problem or a Rubik's cube, pulling chemical structures apart and putting them back together again, in sometimes brilliant ways, finding novel sources and uses for vaccines and drugs in general.

On the good side from a business perspective, pharmaceutical manufacturers often have gaps in manufacturing capacity which simply need to be filled, as a drug may lose market share or patents, for example. Vaccines are a reliable source of growth for the business when other parts of the business such as research and development are not doing so well. But if the research and development are largely outsourced and provided by the government, that makes the business model even better and more profitable.

The government, of course, states they do not fundamentally want to be in the vaccine business. They are simply involved to protect the citizens. The government simply supplies thousands of smart scientists to assist in developing, marketing, and creating guiding principles and protocols for all to follow. Safety is paramount, except when it does not fit with the marketing or advocacy sides of the vaccine business. Where vaccine safety and adverse events may be too difficult to explain to citizens in promotional literature.

As you can see, Vaccine Inc is bigger than any single company. It has its standard players, the government, and their preferred mega vaccine and pharmaceutical manufacturers. Vaccine Inc also has its smaller more flexible players that are ready to jump in whenever needed. As the barrier to entry is not too high, regulations are limited, and legal liability for all players are almost non-existent. The government welcomes all players with open arms and the profit margins are generous all things considered. All players become heroes in a battle against an "invisible enemy", which surely cannot hurt anyone's reputation as being healthcare champions.

Okay, hold on a minute, can these partners just buy into a good reputation based on helping to develop or researching a vaccine? Sure, vaccines are the new "wonder drug" and any manufacturer with capacity can jump right in, and they will magically get a halo over their company's name.

Manufacturers may say, "that's not fair", we are not the government, we are independent, and the government does not control our business. We are separate businesses. The government "regulates us" and does not act as a business partner. The government does, however, share an interest in finding vaccines to help all humankind. Stating "what is good for us, is good for everyone, and we are hard at work finding cures to these devastating illnesses" and "we seek nothing but a small sum for our service to citizens". But if their interest is purely in serving humankind, then why not make your services free or low cost, and ensure the products are safe and free of harm to every person? Okay, enough with the business side of vaccines. I believe it is mostly nonsense, as Vaccine Inc is the government, and the government is in a quasi-public-private partnership with many commercial vaccine interests.

That is how Vaccine Inc was formed and some of the reasoning that went in to formulating a successful partnership of government and private industry in the 1980s. The idea the government wants vaccine companies to do good, and the citizens want access to good and safe vaccines. If they save civilization in the process, then that is even better. A marriage was formed with the noble cause of finding safe and effective vaccines for all citizens. A noble gesture, but as with many marriages, it just does not work exactly as planned.

The Vaccine Inc parties interests often do not align. One party is the controlling party. The other party does not like to be controlled. One party sets up the message to the public. The other party cheats and sets up a relationship with another government. The parties do not share information and facts, making everything a bit dysfunctional. You know, typical marriage issues. You can guess, which party is which, but it simply shows it is mostly a one-sided marriage, with the biggest party controlling the show.

The lies begin and often are little white lies. You know the ones, they will not hurt anyone, and we are in this together to "do good". However, lies lead to more lies, and the parties do not listen as well as time goes by. Each party begins to formulate their own strategies in how to succeed. First they lie to each other, then they begin to lie to the public, so no one knows what the real lie is and what lie is made up to fit a storyline.

Vaccine Inc, the marriage, has kind of evolved in this manner over the last 50 years. I will talk about this later, but for now you should understand our government has adopted steps and controlling interests which are dictated by the government, and its appointed authorities. Vaccine manufacturers are a willing partner in the marriage if the partnership is both financially and mutually interesting.

Where are citizens in this mess of lies? Citizens are a third party, kind of like a consumer looking to a bank, looking for answers and guidance but often just getting false statements as the banker looks to make a profit. Too bad as you should have chosen a better pair as your partners in addressing healthcare strategies. It is unfortunate we must lean on others to make our medical decisions, as we did not take part in the decisions on our own behalf to begin with. To some parties the Vaccine Act sounded like a promising idea, but the law is a mess and offers unbalanced help giving preference to vaccine manufacturers and not citizens.

As a third party, a citizen may look at the bad marriage and simply say, "get divorced", which might be the perfect solution. Or "go to counseling", as one party clearly does not want to bend. From a scientist's perspective, either of these solutions are options for Vaccine Inc, but the likelihood of either party giving in to such an arrangement is greatly limited.

A normal pharmaceutical business could never survive, or even exist, by manufacturing vaccines alone if not for the business subsidies and protections the government gives to vaccine manufacturers. Furthermore, the business model cannot be replicated or changed, as selective enforcement and general protections of the vaccine industry have grown from how Vaccine Inc was created. The Vaccine Act has made the separation of shared interests nearly impossible.

This is how vaccine business is done today. This is not how good and vital drug science is achieved. At some point, a third party must step in and tell the other parties this relationship is not working. In fact, the relationship is kind of toxic for us, the citizens. We all know, vaccines cause both minor and serious injuries, also known as adverse drug reactions, and Vaccine Inc parties do not care to address these concerns, which is a serious problem. It is a problem that has been pushed forward for many decades now, over 35 years, a problem that will not get resolved without meaningful intervention. If left unchecked, the resulting harm could be catastrophic to citizens.

Okay, you say, "but we have not had a major disaster yet". Well we have, but they are mostly smaller disasters managed in smaller settings. In the past, vaccines have been withdrawn from the market because of adverse serious drug reactions and serious adverse complications. Vaccines have also been left in long-term clinical trials with known serious medical complications or side effects. In fact, the manufacturers will often simply withdraw a patient from the clinical study if the patient is found to have a serious medical complication related to the vaccine-related protocol. Even as it may simply be a dosing or metabolic related issue, but for safety reasons, the patient is pulled out of the clinical study, and their data is mostly quashed from further research.

This leaves such discoveries for scientists to research and address, as the vaccine manufacturer has no interest in managing a serious adverse complication, unless there is a clear profitable path giving the manufacturer a marketing edge. Any serious complication will have to wait and can possibly be better understood later when the drug hits the mass market, and the adverse event is further researched for post-marketing reporting after the drug has been approved.

How long does this process for risk discovery, assessment, and action by the manufacturer or FDA take? Well, immediate action would be the desired answer, at least if I were the patient taking a drug, but around 20 to 40 years is a better estimate on timeframe from the moment of discovery of an adverse reaction noted in prominent medical literature to actual reporting by the FDA of a serious adverse drug reaction to medical professionals and the public. This timeframe is for a typical pharmaceutical drug. Vaccine-related adverse event reporting takes quite a bit longer. Somewhere in the 40 to 50-year timeframe on many serious adverse reactions found in post-marketing reports. Vaccine-related adverse event reporting standards are notably held to a much lower standard of required reporting than most drugs.

The process of evaluation falls under the FDA commissioner's window of discretion, a good faith action granted to the FDA commissioner to use his professional instinct and scientific understandings of facts, or to simply make a good faith effort to review and freely interpret the concerns based on some other staff member's opinion and understanding. This is a powerful right when given to any authority, but one many citizens have come to accept as part of our government's selective actions, at virtually every level of government. Science has become less relevant, as we rely on authorities to tell us what the science is rather than trying to understand the science ourselves. Assigned experts look at the science for the citizens and make the decisions simple, so citizens have no need to think but just do as they are told, and no further questions please.

But as I learned in school, please tell me where science facts come from. In science, as in math, a student must rely on logic and laws of nature, and later master algorithms and theorems, injecting speculative and predictive values into problem sets. You can eventually tell what are speculative and what are predictive guesses, like economic statistical modeling, and what are facts as dictated by the laws of math or science. You cannot make such detailed assessments in politics and law. And we must not begin accepting nonsensical speculative science now being put forwarded by authorities and politicians, as history shows citizens have accepted such foolish data and beliefs in the past in many societies which can result in complete catastrophes.

Science does not shift in a crisis. It stays the same. Politics and law shift from moment-to-moment and should not be permitted to override science facts which are true and stated by scientists as observed laws and actions of nature. The discovery of scientific mysteries must be addressed in an open forum for all to investigate and analyze and cannot be based on exclusionary facts derived by select parties or scientists. Lawyers and politicians cannot change logic and science as discretionary actions.

Democracy and transparency of information are taught to citizens as being untouchable principles in our society, and public health and safety are the desired outcomes of such shared values. We do not need to label individuals heroes for simply doing their jobs they selected as a profession. Heroes address problems of great concern and require exceptional effort. In medicine, the need to educate, share facts, and create innovative problem-solving solutions contribute to our success as a profession and a paid service to society. Medical professionals rarely asks our government to find solutions and answers, but simply request our government gives us the resources we need in a crisis to do our jobs, and that all parties are adequately prepared before the crisis to address the needs of the healthcare providers and the public. The government however generally fails in performing its duties to serve citizens in such disasters.

These may seem like deep problems to contemplate, and they are, but they are problems our government prefers not to address jointly with its citizens, for they prefer we let the politicians and authorities give us the answers. They prefer to discuss and address and hopefully resolve our vital concerns, but maybe not right at this very moment, as many will say, "not now, we are too busy". Vaccine Inc is busy suggestively addressing and reallocating resources from our healthcare system, which all parties have neglected for decades. Vaccine Inc does not have time to provide sufficient training and educational resources to medical professionals and the public regarding vaccines. Important vaccine information will be decided and provided to citizens by our government perhaps at some point in the future. And Vaccine Inc is not prepared to manage disaster preparations and recovery, as that falls to the citizens to help each other find answers and solutions. As you might have learned, government problem-solving and actions are not always in our citizens' best interest. Citizen action and individuals caring for our society have always been our greatest strength as a nation.

Vaccine Inc does not properly address vaccine safety concerns. We are in a race against nature, novel viruses and bacteria that will change and grow ever more problematic going forward into the future. Do we count on our government to find discoveries or Vaccine Inc to research and develop safe vaccines at warp speed? Or do we count on science and innovation learned by individuals with deep learned science and thinking freely outside the box? Regardless of which route we chose as a society, there will be sickness, disease, and deaths, but we must choose our battles and follow where history has guided us. Individuals addressing innovative problem solving and solutions to complex problems is a better option when compared to the slow, inefficient, and harmful government options we are often pointed to as our solutions.

Infectious and will surely impact larger populations over a longer period, but what steps shall we take when the government spends trillions of dollars to address a virus that significantly impacts less than 1% of the population? I have heard many times we will have another outbreak like the Spanish flu, but I find little evidence that COVID-19 will be that outbreak. In exchange for some implied protection, Vaccine Inc proposes a vaccine prepared at warp speed (their words, not mine) will help to protect us from this problematic virus.

I suggest there is sufficient evidence of serious adverse risks caused by vaccines in the 1% range of reported adverse vaccine reactions provided by researchers and vaccine manufacturers both in medical literature and post-marketing reporting in many countries. A percentage of these injured patients will become disabled, die, or suffer long-term complications and disabilities. Are we simply trading the implied safeguard of a vaccine, as Vaccine Inc does not address vaccine injuries in a safe tradition? Is the COVID-19 virus a sufficient threat that we must mandate or advocate vaccines as the answer? I suggest the threat of an individual having a vaccine-related injury is not statistically that different from the threat of a COVID-19 or influenza infection causing hospitalization or medical complications, within small percentages stated in statistical reporting.

What should society ask of Vaccine Inc to protect citizens from harm? Many questions have already been asked, many times by scientists, and individuals, and Vaccine Inc continually fails to give answers, failing to make vaccines safer, or provide fair and balanced justice relating to vaccine-related injuries. Vaccine Inc focuses on addressing and pushing the effectiveness narrative, which is easily proven and understood in science. Vaccine Inc openly neglects the safety and adverse risk issues, considering them less important to the public, as they believe the citizens want understood solutions, not understood adverse risks. This has been an issue for decades, and a problem I personally and professionally have addressed in practice and in multiple government agencies and courts. I have learned the lies and false statements made not in one program or agency, but in multiple agencies and courts, and by multiple self-proclaimed experts are the standard public answers. And experts that Vaccine Inc adores and elevates as being higher-level authorities on vaccine messages are the experts they believe are more readily understood and accepted by citizens.

Vaccine Inc promotes and propagandizes vaccines as a solution even as the facts and evidence only demonstrate efficacy, depending on the infection type and behavior of the infectious spread. Perhaps vaccines will slow down the infection spread, but can we not simply slow the disease spread through hygienic practices, quarantine or isolation, and current and future therapeutic protocols? History should be our guide, but we must address them in a safe and efficient drug evaluation process, where safety and effectiveness are given fair analysis by authorities and experts across many fields of science.

Every infectious outbreak in history has resulted in deaths, and COVID-19 has been and will be no different. But should we be rolling the dice and hope a vaccine is the answer, and not another added problem? I would suggest the safety profile for any novel vaccine, like COVID-19, is not adequately developed and in fact the safety profile of many vaccines have been insufficient for decades. Where is the data? And I mean all the data, not bits and pieces of data released as discretionary data to the public. I would suggest all or close to all funding for a COVID-19 vaccine is coming from our government resources. And I will further suggest, much of the COVID-19 vaccine data will be bridged from other vaccines, such as the influenza vaccine. There is simply insufficient time to gather accurate and usable vaccine pharmacological data to properly address any vaccine in such a short window of time.

A gamble with citizens' health? Yes, Vaccine Inc takes the gamble every year with patients' health and will willingly gamble with the citizen's health in promoting a COVID-19 vaccine. It is not a noble-gesture type transaction but a business transaction. Many parties ask for the vaccine, and if you are the United States government, the government generally gives citizens what they ask for using simple terms like public health, protection of citizens and vital actions needed for the national defense against "invisible" enemies they cannot see and do not understand. These blurred actions have backfired in the past, and you can look to our military who are our loyal test subjects on many of our drugs, as well as many countries that provide research and clinical studies to find answers to such concerns.

The risks of adverse side effects caused by any vaccine may be limited, or they could be great. And the patients that bear the greatest impact may be the population that can least afford to be impacted. The poor and disadvantaged, many ethnic citizens, and citizens with ongoing medical conditions. A suggested risk of managing an infection in some patients is simply a suggested reason to widely vaccinate selected segments of the population. If the medical condition worsens, doctors often prefer to deal with the medical condition worsening. Patients however should demand information to ensure any drug is right for the individual citizen's health situation, and an understanding that complications are manageable and comprehended as adverse events related to vaccines.

Patients often misunderstand their rights to be informed and their right to make the final decision of informed consent. Many patients simply look at the doctor and say, "well you have the syringe in your hand, you make the decision", as doctors are in some fashion the more informed person in making a medical decision. That argument is fair but is not correct. The only time a doctor can make a final decision is if it is life or death, and all reasonable medical options available have been tried. Patients are always in control of their own health and should always look for and demand information before they give permission to any medical provider to make a medical decision for them. Learn the facts, process the facts, and make your medical decisions based on the facts. Simple steps to live by.

I personally have concerns with being an early adopter of any drug or procedure that may on the surface have enticingly noted few risks, but also have many misunderstood and not fully expected adverse events, commonly called adverse drug reactions. This problem happens with all commercial products, and there is a big difference between an electronic gadget that does not work as advertised and a drug that does not work as advertised. Again, I refer you back to liability, and the safety net our federal and state governments imply vaccines have as a general consumer protection. The safety nets offered for vaccines are however exceedingly poor and often fail to assist vaccine-injured citizens. The Vaccine Injury Compensation Program (the VICP) suggested as the safety net for vaccine injuries managed by our government is rigged in the vaccine's favor, and not in a small way, but in an exceptionally large way. I say "vaccine" as a claim for injury is not a claim for settlement with vaccine manufacturers or medical professionals, but a claim seeking settlement from a biased government specialty court. You can read the rules of the court online at https://www.hrsa.gov/vaccine-compensation or searching for and reading the Vaccine Act. I understood the rules, but I did not understand the shifty practices of lawyers who manipulate the rules of the court. The VICP program permits discretion and countermeasures, acts by the Secretary of Health and Human Services (HHS), to address injuries, but these actions are in general discretionary actions that can harm citizens injured by a vaccine.

To put the vaccine concern into tech-speak, which may be easier to understand, this should be a stop and hard reboot moment. Proceed at your own risk. Consider all actions final. All future function and benefits of a vaccine decision being made may seriously impact future functionality of your body. This action is not reversible and will possibly lead to further disability and loss of use. Is this your final determination to go ahead? Okay, now we can proceed and vaccinate. What do you do when these messages pop-up on your computer screen? Again, as with your computer, you can choose to do as you like. But a hard drive is much easier to replace than an injured body.

Are certain populations more impacted by the COVID-19 virus and should be immunized first or in large test groups? I do not know; in fact, I doubt anyone knows today. Just keep in mind if you are first in line, you are also the first test group of a mass-supplied novel drug, which has both benefits and risks. I suggest citizens know the risks or at least discuss the risks with a knowledgeable medical professional with knowledge of vaccines specifically. If your doctor or pharmacist is not sure, or simply point to a CDC guideline or statement, or promotional poster, ask for more information. Or simply make an "informed" choice and give an informed consent based on a most-likely uninformed wager. What those risks and responses are will likely not be known for years, maybe decades.

Vaccine researchers and immunologists know some of these risks but will generally overlook them as they affect so few patients. I suggest you ask the challenging questions, as the questions will not be answered by the VICP special master who have limited knowledge and understanding of the science. The VICP court trial is more of a popularity contest among experts, except the government has a much bigger "expert" population to draw from. In the case for my son, I matched a Father of Immunology (a very high distinction given to specialists in the field of Immunology by other immunologists) to argue against a distinguished Nephrologist (who the VICP special master and government decided to elevate the government's expert to being a Patriarch of Nephrology, an equally high distinction but not granted by his own fellow professionals, and granted as a discretion by the special master in the case, as she did not want him to feel small or anything, despite being thoroughly embarrassed by his own testimony). The special master was easily confused by the science, and legal discussions led into nonsensical science discussions, which I will talk about later in the book. Or you can read the VICP court transcript online on my website and draw your own conclusions.

I firmly believe today an average citizen would not stand a chance in the VICP court, and I can say multiple parties including the Secretary of HHS, the FDA commissioner, the court judges and many other authorities overseeing our vaccine programs are simply unconcerned authorities, and would not stand a chance in submitting a vaccine injury claim that is not on the Vaccine Injury Table. A Vaccine Table injury is a limited set of injuries found on a matrix created by VICP authorities after the Vaccine Act was adopted into law. Off-Table claims (vaccine-related injuries not in the matrix) are aggressively contested by the Department of Justice who function as attorneys defending the Secretary of Health and Human Services. And no, the citizens never get to meet the Secretary, and the Secretary never even has to make a statement, just serves as the authority making an appearance by name on the injured party's legal claim against Vaccine Inc. The claim may as well be You vs. the U.S. Government, or You vs. the World. This is not an argument against the vaccine or the manufacturer, but an argument against Vaccine Inc, who again is our government. Get ready for crazy town because few are ready for this much craziness and bogus science dragged on for years and years. Or to shorten the claims process go directly to an offer of settlement which will likely be an unacceptably low and insufficient offer to cover the impact of the vaccine-related injury and certainly will not follow any other federal guidelines with regards to appropriate settlement actions. Yes, in case you did not know, there are Federal Guidelines for Fair Settlement on the books, with specific guidance on what is fair and appropriate in settling litigation with our government.

Just do not expect anyone in the VICP court or working for the DOJ to follow these rules or guidelines. As it is more like, how is the judge feeling today? Not good, well sorry for you that is too bad, maybe we should try to see what the judge is thinking on a different day. In my son's case, the special master sought to validate her junior-high school level nurse friend with combined poor medical, math, and financial skills that she pulled in to help develop a settlement offer for a lifetime of medical care needs relating to my son's vaccine injury. But the nurse and the special master's financial and medical skills clearly did not align with the guidelines noted as "the right thing to do" according to the Vaccine Act's legislated intent. The nurse's life care plan made some odd projections of future medical and care costs clearly based on improperly developed cost estimates pulled out of thin air or perhaps some government welfare cost book that sat decades old somewhere, not an actual cost estimate requested from the facility the nurse suggested as being her recommended guide for making cost estimates.

We sat ready to show actual costs from multiple care facilities, including the nurse's stated recommended facility, which she lied to us as being verified but learned was entirely fabricated. But the special master was unconcerned by our more expert detailed cost facts, the special master simply stood firm and demanded acceptance of a vague and undetermined settlement as a take-it-or-leave-it offer. Her long-term favored nurse friend served as her basis in demanding acceptance of a settlement, but her friend also failed to do her government-contracted job to prepare a real-life care plan. This is how the VICP operates today, not how the law was legislated or enacted as a fair law in 1986, as the VICP extended the Law to include a matrix table of acceptable injuries caused by vaccines which became part of the program's redesigned rules in the mid-1990s.

The VICP program gradually shifted from being a suggestively fair compensation vaccine program to becoming a biased vaccine-endorsement support program. The lawyers administering the VICP program changed the rules and framework of the Vaccine Law with little legislative discussion, and zero-found citizen discussion. A fatal and flawed action endorsed by many parties in Vaccine Inc as the best option for protecting both the vaccine manufacturers and the government funding resources. An example of an aggressive action taken against patients that are harmed by vaccine-related injuries where such injuries have since 1986 become mostly a discretionary afterthought.

Perhaps, citizens believe this is a matter for the lawyers and politicians to settle. But the Vaccine court's VICP Bar, lawyers approved to represent claimants, are fatally limited in number, as most lawyers who are in practice in the VICP bar are limited in skills and knowledge of vaccine injuries, except when they can argue a substantial payout for their services inside their own head. Vaccine Table injuries are the easiest to resolve in time and effort, and a relatively easy payout, as the court compensates all legal and expert fees regardless of outcome. There are few substantial arguments needed for a listed Vaccine Table injury, which simply requires filing a claim and settling the claim's costs for future costs and medical care which requires little effort and the payout to the attorney of record, and can easily be paid out as $50,000 or more. Make the arguments a little more challenging, and the payout to an attorney grows to over several hundreds of thousands of dollars. And the promised payout to the injured party is often nominal at best and take-it-or-leave-it, or the special master can decide the injured party will get zero. It is a game of craps where the dice and results are rigged. All claims and costs decided and paid out by another member of the same shady profession, lawyers. The government has made the lawyers work for their pay, but in the end, the lawyers ALWAYS get paid, as it is a defined requirement in the Vaccine Act.

This book will cover many of these issues, and I simply ask you to read my concerns and to ask questions. You have a right to demand vaccine safety and facts, which I suggest this action as your best choice. I expected our government to be smarter, and to give science a fair shake, and to get the scientific facts right. It was an error on my part for believing we have a fair and just legal system.

Who knows? I know the government freely makes many empty promises to address their flawed preferred vaccine programs. Some promises are suggested as being valid, but citizens must be vigilant, as they will not get a fair hearing regarding most vaccine injuries in the VICP if you ever have a vaccine injury that reaches this level of argument as a claim. Many citizens confuse drug liability and vaccine liability laws, along with most every day general and "expert" lawyers who often get facts and vaccine court rules wrong. Vaccine laws are federal laws and follow distinctly different, but not overly complex, statutes and rules. There are virtually no state vaccine laws, as the federal Vaccine Act is the absolute vaccine law of our nation. Any thoughts of filing a small claim, or local claim are mostly mute. All vaccine injury claims must generally go through the VICP. And your limits to file are restricted by time limits, which a VICP lawyer can help you determine if you are eligible but may or may not help you get through the claim process. Vaccine Bar approved attorneys know the law but often fail to understand the science or injury mechanisms and openly reject complex cases. I wish I could do that as a medical professional, just send me the easy customers with no problems or complaints. Who said an attorney is always mandated to advocate for their clients? We all know that is a lie, and always has been. What a poor excuse for a profession, lawyers.

I can argue the science endlessly and I am sure the vaccine medical experts with a vested interest in vaccines would argue the value of vaccines as a drug, but my arguments are not just safety-related judgement calls and what you believe you can do personally to protect your family. My arguments are foundational and unwavering beliefs in our constitutional rights. It is essential that we demand our rights to make choices, and that we demand information with evidence and facts relating to adverse vaccine reported facts. It is essential that we have information as citizens and as medical professionals treating all citizens who must be given complete and correct data and facts to share with our patients.

I do not need condensed, dumbed-down data and statements of how vaccine things work. But as many citizens say, I need hard-science facts and evidence. I also suggest we have many therapeutic choices that are current and have already undergone stringent clinical trials and post-approval reporting including pharmacovigilant studies and case reports regarding verified safety concerns. Not that these protocols do not present a risk or medical concerns, but the risks are defined, and the risks have liability for mandating both pharmacovigilance and vigorous reporting as the medical professionals have a legal interest in all harm that may be done to all patients. All drugs have these types of drug reporting standards and liability, except for vaccines.

The government and Vaccine Inc has had their time, more time than should have been granted by citizens, to be upfront and honest with the people of the United States. More than thirty years of time in fact. Other governments have been far more upfront and compelling in addressing vaccine safety concerns of many vaccines. If you support the idea of having vaccine drug information withheld from citizens, you can stop reading here. If you would like more information, I will gladly open my records. Records which are secret to the public, but not sealed. In fact, they belong to me, as I was the claimant party of record and they are my records. The public has no access to these records, except through me. VICP Bar attorneys will not give up these records for fear of retribution by the special masters and judges. The courts act as if the records are sealed for some twisted form of privacy, but they are not. Some claimants cannot get their VICP lawyers to give up their records, but the records belong to the client, not the attorney. I believe I am one of the few, if not only, claimants to ever offer to open their court records completely to the public to review and decide for themselves. Who is the bigger fool? Me or the courts, or maybe that is a loaded question.

The public currently gets the sterile and filtered decisions of judges, which can be a stupid opinion of a special master and judges as reference to misunderstood facts and evidence. Too bad the judges and special masters cannot even remember the facts right, but maybe I can change that. Maybe future claims will reference actual testimony and evidence as referenced to facts, rather than nonsensical memories of aging special masters and judges. I will give you the unfiltered facts and opinions of the court records and statements by me and my opinions and references to facts which are supported by science and evidence you may find shocking. Or maybe citizens support and like the VICP program the way it is now, or believe it is the way citizens believe our justice system should be? The VICP has failed to properly administer the legislated program for citizens for decades now, why not carry on for a few more decades or centuries so we can see if any more citizens can catch on to this fake court system of fake justice and science? My records and supporting reference material will be available online to review.

The legal aspects of my case for my son are now mute arguments, as a disabled citizen was given no legal representation or fair assistance as required under the ADA law to address an unjust vaccine claim process filed against our government. The Supreme Court is the end of the road, and they had no interest in hearing facts and evidence, even suggesting the government's experts acting as the voice of the government are permitted to lie and perjure themselves shamelessly for the protection of vaccines, without any fear of being reprimanded or punished. I know, it happens all the time, right? In fact, it happens more often than you may expect in the VICP Court as it is only two steps from the Supreme Court. The Supreme Court Justices simply have no interest in addressing vaccine matters. They defer these issues to Congress, and we all know how competent our congressional representatives are in getting things done. And the President, the President could step in, but unfortunately, we do not ever have a President with any scientific and pharmaceutical knowledge other than perhaps as an investor. Some Presidential candidates make suggestive political statements of vaccine injury concerns then make a 180-degree turn when in office, which is very odd how politicians' flip-flops match the flip-flops of government experts who change their position on-the-fly with a few extra bucks in their pocket. This seemingly leaves corrective actions to the citizens, the citizens must act to protect themselves, as our government is largely incompetent regarding vaccine safety related concerns specifically, but also regarding many drugs, which are endorsed and poorly managed by an otherwise biased set of drug and vaccine regulatory and guidance agencies.

My child was a victim of our vaccine law and the VICP program. I am passionate about my son, and I will always assist my son; but I also fear for many citizens that have no such support or medical knowledge. Can you as a regular citizen afford to make the wrong choice? Can you afford to let our government and Vaccine Inc make the wrong choices for you or your loved ones? Are you prepared to address these concerns? Because the government is certainly not prepared to assist citizens. If you are prepared to make the choice, or give that choice away, just understand it was your choice. Some would suggest it is the American way. I would suggest it is a foolish choice to answer to a foolish Law, which citizens must learn and understand before accepting any vaccination.

As a final statement here, I must state I am a scientist, a pharmacist, and a patriot. I have genuine concerns for all citizens, and passionately believe our government is acting outside our individual interests. Together as citizens we can address vaccine safety concerns and a flawed vaccine program by mandating change to our Vaccine Law which must be consistent with our values and recognize all harm that can affect individuals. I suggest all citizens should review and understand the Vaccine Act and should independently determine the Law is flawed beyond any suggested repair or replacement and must be scrapped as a Law that is unsound and harmful to citizens. To be fair, all drugs are drugs and must be treated equally, and all injuries that impact citizens must be treated accurately with scientific facts and evidence presented as a drug concern to our government. If drugs known as vaccines are to be mandated and declared safe, I suggest it is proper to eliminate the Vaccine Act, and let the chips fall where they may, but citizens should also understand the government will not let that happen. Our government has the backs of Vaccine Inc members covered, but not the citizen's back when a real injury occurs. Just keep that thought in the back of your mind, as you are asked to make an informed consent decision for not just one vaccine, but many vaccines going forward into the future. To learn and understand more, simply read on.

CHAPTER 2

A Brief History Regarding Plagues, Pandemics, and other Public Health Concerns...

I start here as many readers may be familiar with the history of infectious disease outbreaks, but for those that are unfamiliar I offer a brief history in social struggles with plagues, pandemics and infections that have impacted humans. Plagues, pandemics, epidemics, and various disease outbreaks have devastated the lives of people resulting in death, pain and suffering, and causing enormous economic impact for many millenniums, dating back to before the earliest days of recorded disease history. The tracking and recording of plagues and pandemics have improved in the last few centuries, primarily following the Black Plagues of the Middle Ages, which ran from around 1334 to around 1800, but other documented plague-type outbreaks have occurred from 3500 BC all the way up to today.

Yes, the bacteria that caused the Black Plague has been reported in many locations globally in 2020. The Black Plague from the Middle Ages is thought to have been caused by the bacterium *Yersinia pestis* (generally labelled *Y. pestis*). Pandemics are a continuing infectious concern, but bacterial plagues are not as much of a concern today as the availability of antibiotics and infectious treatment protocols have greatly improved from the days of the early Black Plague. In fact, many infectious outbreaks have become less problematic since the discovery of penicillin in 1928. But a concern has developed recently as bacteria have developed more antibiotic-resistance and are evolving into "superbugs", which are less responsive to current antibiotics. Today, *Y. pestis,* the bacteria that caused the Black Plague is generally isolated by medical professionals and is treated with antibiotics, so *y. pestis* outbreaks are less of a general population concern. Many superbug-type infections are now the more difficult infections to treat. Do we have a vaccine for *y. pestis*? No, because there are antibiotic therapeutic treatment options, and the infectious disease is not widespread. How about some of the other superbugs? Again, no, as vaccines have not been developed to address all infectious pathogens. Most bacterial infections that have caused major outbreaks in the past are now treatable with antibiotics. And antivirals are picking up as a therapeutic viral infection treatment tool, but antiviral drugs do not work quite like antibiotics. They slow down viral growth, where a patient's immune system still must do a lot of the work. Bacterial and viral infection treatments are not the same, but these types of infections are often linked as causes of primary and secondary infections in many patients, where the infections can be occurring at the same time or sequentially. Parasites, like worms and fungal infections can also be dangerous as antiparasitic and antifungal drug treatments are available but are also limited, and the infections are often either quite simple or extraordinarily complex to treat depending on location of the infecting parasite. Most doctors do not address parasite and fungal infections inside the body often until the infection has moved to a more advanced stage, as the symptoms may be less obvious in the early stages of infection.

The word plague has been used in some current discussions related to COVID-19, but COVID-19 is not a plague and references should be eliminated from the current discussion as we are not having a plague. What we have today is a viral pandemic based on an infectious disease caused by a coronavirus. Viruses are not treated by antibiotics, but may be treated by antivirals, which is a newer class of pharmaceutical agents. Antibiotics may also be used to treat development of a secondary bacterial infection, often caused by clinical complications such as inflammation and excess mucus related to the primary viral infection which can lead to a bacterial infection, as bacteria love this type of growth media for development inside the body. A primary viral infection, like COVID, may be the setup punch, and the secondary infections can become the knockout punch. In general, most viral infections are treated as an unaccompanied infection, and are often treatable depending on other complicating factors and a patient's general health. Viral infections can be serious, but supportive treatments are often sufficient in returning the patient back to good health. The virus class causing COVID-19 is called a Severe Acute Respiratory Syndrome Coronavirus 2 (SARS-CoV-2). Sometimes confused by citizens, bacterial and viral infections are not the same, as bacterial cells cause slightly different infections than viral strains. A viral infection is generally a single RNA strand that infect human cells and can be very disruptive to cell functions.

As stated above, many people also confuse the terms plagues, pandemic and epidemic, or a simple infectious disease outbreak. A plague is a widespread outbreak related to a bacterial or viral source. It is generally thought the Black Plague was primarily caused by y. *pestis*, but various other bacterium or viruses may have also played a role in plague cycles, including the Black Plague. The general understanding of the Black Plague spread was related to the bacteria transmitted through fleas on rats in trade ships from port-to-port and then over land after infecting the port city's citizens. Many infectious disease outbreaks are related to spread of diseases linked by trade, exploration, war, and movement of populations from one location to the other regions. In today's world, global spread is common as many infectious diseases spread easily as global trade and international business are common practices. Infectious diseases are closely monitored world-wide. A true plague-type outbreak has not been seen in the U.S. since the discovery of antibiotics, but some areas of impoverished regions of the world still experience some forms of plague, which despite the scary name are generally treatable but often occur in populations with poor healthcare resources and limited personnel to manage the outbreaks.

An epidemic is different from the plague and is defined as a rapid spread of an infectious disease to a large segment of the population in a defined area within a short period of time. A pandemic is an epidemic of a specific infectious disease that spreads across larger regions and affects a large group of people on many continents which is generally defined as a worldwide spread. An endemic infectious disease is smaller, usually only impacting smaller groups of people, and is generally not considered a pandemic. An example of an endemic disease is a common recurring seasonal influenza outbreak, where the number of infected people are generally more stable which can occur simultaneously in multiple regions of the world but are not necessarily spread worldwide. Our current infectious outbreak of COVID-19 is considered a pandemic because it has spread globally across most regions of the earth impacting many widespread populations. The word pandemic does not necessarily imply a more serious infection but can have an effect on a larger group of people. All infectious diseases in general can involve serious medical complications and progression of sickness up to and including death.

In general, COVID-19, which is again a viral infection, has had a marked impact on specific age groups generally noted as significantly impacting the elderly in all regions globally. The impact of COVID-19 on children and otherwise healthy individuals has often been nominal with notably fewer serious cases and complications reported. The general guidance at this point follows the logic elderly citizens have a more limited immune system and have few or no antibodies developed to fight the COVID-19 virus. Healthy children and adults have a relatively robust immune system and appear to be less likely to be impacted by exposure to the COVID pathogen. The other groups suggested as being impacted are those with pre-existing medical conditions, which implies a significant large percentage of the population, as the authorities suggest individuals with asthma, high blood pressure, diabetes, obesity, immunocompromised medical conditions, and other medical conditions are at higher risk of a complication related to all infectious diseases. There is some science here to support these claims of impact to these groups of patients, but much of the concern applied to this group is speculative and may be tied to drug treatments and/or the underlying medical complications related to the pre-existing condition. Other suggested risks of infection are the higher incident and impact felt among certain ethnic groups, but this too is speculative, as infectious diseases are rarely genetic specific. Suggested racial differences are more likely related to poor healthcare programs, poor government administration of healthcare services, and general differences in cultural practices regarding social distancing. In other words, infectious diseases are not commonly considered a race issue, but are more closely tied to communal and personal hygiene practices. There is limited science to support genetic impact tied to a few infectious pathogens, but such differences are generally small, where treatments and outcomes if treated properly should result in the same outcomes among all citizen regardless of race.

Another area of current concern is testing, and while testing has improved in relationship to many past infectious outbreaks, infectious disease testing is still poor and almost non-existent in many regions of the world. Testing accuracy is not perfect, and generally hovers around 60-80% accuracy in surface swab testing, which is considered adequate by many. Blood testing is more accurate, but also takes more time and resources not readily available in many locations. At some point in time, most of the population will likely test positive for having developed antibodies or having had exposure to the COVID-19 virus, as it is a highly contagious pathogen, similar in spread to other viruses like the viruses that cause the common cold, which is also highly contagious. Currently, the testing locations and population groups being tested are widespread and provide poor statistical data for analysis, as testing results are broad-scoped and difficult to interpret, which leads to many speculative statements and poorly stated concerns. Do not feel ashamed if you have not been tested for COVID-19. Many individuals have been exposed to the COVID-19 virus and have not been tested yet. Current testing procedures are not the best diagnostic tools but are simply one of the few diagnostic tools available to isolate and quarantine patients based on real science. Other diagnostic clinical tools are related to patients developing clinical symptoms of a COVID infection, which acts primarily as a guide for treating symptoms but is not really a proper test for COVID-19.

Epidemiologists are the scientists who collect and analyze distribution patterns of diseases of all types, which includes both infectious diseases and noninfectious diseases, with a higher priority given to infectious diseases. Statistical reporting standards for analysis are defined by national and global standards, but citizens should understand reporting in general is local and relies on the training of the local reporting staff. Epidemiology and public health reporting positions are newer professions developed to track health trends which are significantly influenced by the federal government, as epidemiology reporting and training is largely government funded. As stated previously, COVID-19 is currently listed as the primary medical complication relating to hospitalizations, so even as other medical complications may consist of a prominent comorbidity that can often lead to death or hospitalization, which may be serious alone or in combination with any infection, COVID is the reported primary cause for medical complications. Pneumonia-Influenza-Coronavirus (also called PIC) infections are routinely listed as the primary risk for epidemiological reporting, especially for causes of death or hospitalization. In broad statistical reporting this can distort short-term statistical data, as more in-depth analysis is deficient and is often not studied until many years later, or can be simply overlooked as not being relevant to having an immediate need for analysis. Sketchy testing and sketchy reporting do not equal good science, but these practiced methods of statistical analysis are in the early stages of being learned relative to the history of infectious disease studies and suggest utilizing excellent information technology to collect and sort data as being useful in future projections and analysis. At some point in the future, the analysis of data for science is sure to be more relevant as more data usually equals better results. The quality and quantity of useful statistical data is just not the current practiced standard. Citizens should not look to government reports and statistical data for relevance to absolute trends, but to local and isolated regional trends.

History is the guide we must follow and where we must learn lessons from, and history also dictates how we allocate our resources as a society. Many authorities suggest patients who die or are hospitalized from an infectious disease would not have died or been hospitalized if not for the infection. Breaking down important data and determining which needed resources are lacking takes a lot of time to analyze. The data is wrapped into private and public databases and is usually buried from public access for years. These facts matter as citizens rely on obscure data and evidence to understand obscure facts, like why the U.S. leads all nations in reported COVID-19 cases, and several individual states are exceptionally out of normal range for cases reported. The answers can be obvious, as many areas have more testing which would obviously equal more cases reported, and other deviations may never be fully understood as the data does not provide ample data. Current speculative assumptions are sometimes good and are sometimes way off-base in terms of being related to the scientific evidence offered up for analysis.

The statistical data matters on the medical side mostly relating to allocation of resources, as medical professionals report needs for resources and the need to develop best protocols based on available resources. If there is for example an antibiotic shortage, other therapeutic treatment options must be assessed. This too is a local concern and a funding concern, as the government and insurance companies often apply cost caps, which the government can override, but does not change the fact there are shortages. Shortages are often related to government and manufacturer decisions linked to efforts to lower drug costs, which is a balancing act driven mostly by federal authorities and legislated actions. And in today's world, are aligned with which drugs are most cost effective and result in the shortest hospital stays in deciding which treatment plan of action is most favored. History shows us resources and trained professionals often mark a successful campaign against any infectious outbreak. Yet government authorities do not seem to understand how that relates to decreased resources, shortages of drugs, and many medical professionals being underutilized or inappropriately utilized relative to their skills in an infectious outbreak. This again is related to the government's failure to make good healthcare decisions relating to resources and need to provide appropriate levels of healthcare services and care uniformly to all citizens during an infectious outbreak.

The time-honored policy of documenting and identifying infectious diseases started centuries ago in early civilization, customarily by theorists and mathematicians who tried to apply some logic to the diseases and ailments. The distinguished practice of making observations continued for centuries reflecting the general concerns of rulers and religious leaders often dictating which social practices were most favored to protect their rule. For many centuries, the most common infectious disease transcribers worked for leaders of the church, for example monks, and the cause of many illnesses and diseases were attributed to being acts of God. Infectious disease documentation methods picked up the pace in the 1800s and really accelerated in the 1900s. Computers and technology have helped analyze the recent data, but while the art of statistics and data are helpful in analyzing the spread of the diseases, it is simply not a perfect art or science at this point in time.

Today, we still see data which has been exploited to make short-term projections and estimations, and guessing which statistical model is best has become more of a game than a science. Government officials and politicians today make errors in trusting statistical models and projections, much like past leaders trusted and gave support to less scientific guesses and ideas. Today, many non-medically trained authorities suggest another Spanish flu-type pandemic is imminent. The Spanish flu caused hundreds of millions of deaths globally, whereas COVID-19 is nowhere near the severity of the Spanish flu.

Therapeutic drugs and clinical tools have been greatly improved since the 1918 Spanish flu outbreak. But as in all modern-era infectious disease outbreaks, all forms of media broaden the infectious narrative to capture public interest and to grab viewers' attention, which is a journalistic tactic used to gain influence and profit for centuries. In fact, the evolution of journalism has paralleled the evolution of politics and infectious disease treatments as tools used to manipulate the public's immediate concerns. Add newer available social media, and the pieces to a perfect storm of misinformation and disinformation exist, but who should we trust for better information, our government? Our government is not the best source for honest information, as nongovernment-based resources often offer better data and resources to discovery and learn science and facts and are more readily available for citizens to access.

New technology and classical sciences will be instrumental in pushing forward and understanding up-to-date science, but citizens must be wary of authorities and scientists that wish to skewer facts to fit their preferred narrative rather than providing scientific proofs and facts. Many authorities, especially politicians, love science filtered through some preferred set of narratives, which are slanted to fit the narrative they prefer to be relevant but are not fully supported by scientific evidence. For many, science is not science, but a method to influence the many citizens who do not understand science. Often in ways that benefit the authorities or grants power and wealth to the scientists who hold titles and designated positions as being of higher importance than everyday citizens.

Citizens will be told "science is science, and we must follow the science"; but we must also be cautious in which parties are providing the science, as science has a clear and learned method which requires documentation and not just nonsensical statements from a few authorities and scientists. Such statements may be partially correct but also require scientific verification. Science, as in medicine, requires concepts and products be theorized, evaluated, retested, and conclusions must be made from the observed evidence. Facts can be learned as understood science needing further evaluation or eventually with verification are declared laws of nature. Conclusions of science facts can often be speculative or misstated until full facts are understood but should be noted as understood concerns until rejected by scientists using the same testing methods and standards. So, a logical conclusion to a noted scientific observation cannot be dismissed, without fully explaining the observed science through other mechanisms of learned science. Many scientific observations often reported as a case report are expressed as significant discoveries but also require a need for added research to fully understand the science. Scientists set the threshold for addressing these spontaneous discoveries, but governments often provide the funding for research and control the level of funding for such research, and often apply pressure to scientists to control predetermined conclusions which may later be proven as false.

Citizens should never trust a scientist or group of scientists that present false facts and then try to cover up their science with claims that the science is declared valid simply because they are the experts and they state the facts without any further discussion or reference to other scientific evidence or proofs by their scientific peers. This is a common error of experts who do not appreciate the requirement of reporting valid science facts using proper scientific arguments. Many experts often make flawed scientific statements and errors. Where the facts should be challenged with requests for referenced data, studies, or sources used by the experts to verify the facts. In many cases, there are none, or are facts poorly reviewed by other scientists, which often go decades or even centuries before being proven incorrect. Again, look to the Middle Ages where plagues and pandemics were attributed to God's punishment, or the astrological position of the stars, or earthquakes and weather changes. The science was lacking, and simply because the science was not understood by the scientists-of-the-day, many citizens agreed to these nonsensical arguments of causation of infectious diseases, as bacteria and viruses were not yet discovered. Science was held back, as religious leaders had a self-serving interest to maintain power over citizens. For if citizens cannot observe and document the science then citizens cannot understand the science, so one must only create a logical explanation the common citizen will accept as a cause based on false science. Today, as more and more science has become available and accessible to scientists worldwide, it is now necessary to address science and facts which are observed and documented by many scientists, and not from the standpoint of authorities and professions who argue philosophy and politics, but by professions that argue science. If a scientific fact is reported and documented, such facts cannot be dismissed as being rare and insignificant. These facts must be studied and explained as they are important discoveries which can lead to other discoveries and ultimately answers to scientific questions not presently fully understood.

As citizens, we consistently want answers and solutions, even when answers and solutions are not straightforward. That is part of human nature. The need to be informed and to be given choices. While we do not have all the answers about infectious diseases, we do have knowledge of what medical professionals can and cannot do to address infectious disease uncertainties. Many human infections are bacterial in origin and are treatable with antibiotics. Yet, bacteria change and adapt making many antibiotics less useful over time. Or in other instances, antibiotic ingredients become less readily available without delay and are controlled by select companies, which increases the monetary value of the drugs, but causes widespread harm to humanity as the antibiotics become less available to treat all citizens. Citizens remain uninformed of critical drug concerns and authorities jump in to address these concerns and make choices of which medical options are best to address the growing problems for society. These choices are often poor choices made for citizens by authorities.

Who do we blame for poor choices? Historically, we blame government leaders, politicians, and the drug manufacturers for mismanagement and making important business decisions based on self-interests and profits rather than serving citizens. Pharmaceutical and medical profiteering practices have always been an evolving issue and has grown worse since the beginning of modern pharmaceutical and medical capitalism, which interestingly parallels the promotional practices of vaccines. Business decisions and practices often play key roles in management of infectious outbreaks. Politicians and media again often play a role in spinning who the guilty parties are, but these bands of suggestive influencers rarely offer solutions or methods for resolving the conflicts in science. Greed is a powerful cause for misstatements of science, but so is the feeling of power and importance sensed by those making the often-flawed statements.

Citizens should learn their lessons from history. From the early days of history, citizens quickly realized the need to isolate and quarantine away from infected humans and animals, which was a normal and instinctual early learned safety practice to stay healthy. Later humans learned to sterilize and use good hygienic practices, which again were good, but these practices only took centuries to understand, as societies evolved from using streets and common areas for sanitation purposes. Addressing these concerns were eventually understood to slow the spread of infection or at least keep the infection isolated to a few groups of citizens, where less desirable citizens were often given poorer conditions to live in and survive. Crude evaluations of medical treatments and the availability of safe drug therapeutic treatments follow a similar path today, where the best solutions are often applied to the few select citizens deemed worthy, and others must simply adapt. Preventative measures like low-cost sanitizing products and later vaccines were pushed as the low-cost solution to manage infectious diseases more widely.

The history of infectious diseases has documented large numbers of deaths, sometimes deaths from widespread plagues, such as The Black Plague where deaths exceeded 50% of the world's population. No one was spared, all age groups and all societies in general suffered equally. Wealth and knowledge had little influence as the infections were not always spread person-to-person. In the Black Plague, it was spread from flea to rat to food and surfaces to humans. Most infections are mostly unseen and are misunderstood by citizens. You would think today with improved technology we would be in better shape of informing citizens, but in reality it is a long learning process to collect data and analyze trends to understand the characteristics and behaviors of a microorganism, and the proper medical steps needed to address the infectious pathogen. We are years ahead of earlier outbreaks, but we still practice the same poorly evolved practices and steps for preparation of outbreaks.

During the early plagues, ships with a sick crew were banned from many ports; or as one city became overwhelmed with disease, nearby city-states would shutoff access to outsiders. The key steps to managing the outbreak often taken by leaders was to isolate the infected citizens and banish select individuals and their families. Segments of the population were left to independently find a path to survival often with limited assistance by other citizens or societal resources. And, if they somehow survived, they were surely blessed. As many believed the diseases were in some way acts of God, everyone should pray, and pray a lot, as most believed plagues were punishment for their sins and ungodly actions.

Real science was not freely discovered in this era as the age of medical and life sciences did not begin until later centuries. Scientists in the days of the early plagues pointed to understood observable sciences as signs of cause for the infectious diseases. These were the sciences of the times, and of course if you collapsed and fell sick, well surely that was a bad thing for the fallen victim's family. As the disease began to spread, everyone would go into isolation and small groups took care of each other except for the kings, religious leaders, and nobles, and elites who demanded exceptional care and isolation. It is somewhat odd that as much as science has changed, with emphasis on scientific methods, the application of science and social needs practices have largely stayed the same.

Which citizens are most important to a society, and at what critical costs should all citizens pay to save their lives? Are some applications of science worth more than other applications? History often shows us that leaders and elite citizens claim exception, but at what cost? Often it is at the cost of poorer citizens and the children. These are philosophical arguments and historically have pointed to leaders and nobles acting as Noble Liars. A noble lie is an untruth or falsely stated fact or set of facts knowingly announced by an elite individual or voice for a government stated to maintain collective harmony or to advance a stated agenda. The noble lie is a philosophical concept originated by Plato as described in his book the *Republic*. Where noble and elite citizens simply lie to the masses, as they simply believe they must tell lies and falsehoods to the uninformed less intelligent citizens to save society and declare harmony over chaos.

These lies are commonly used to advance a particular agenda, like today the agenda promoting everyone should get vaccinated as all vaccines are "perfectly safe", but leaves the individuals to struggle for answers to adverse vaccine reactions and injuries on their own. Noble liars may express empathy and concern but are generally insincere in their concerns for individuals. This concept of confronting Noble Liars is one of the foundational philosophies which led to the formation of democratic nations. The desires of men to seek self-governance and manifest destiny, separating facts and evidence from false statements of Noble Liars. Every individual should choose their own destiny. Addressing Noble Liars and false leaders is a concern all citizens must address as shared interests for all citizens of democracies.

CHAPTER 3

...More Infectious Disease History. Just Because.

Apothecary (early pharmacy) specialists were the earliest medical profession to offer elixirs and chemicals from herbs and other sources, which included many early anti-infectives that were effective in treating infectious diseases but also were known to be harmful, and even deadly. Chemists (or apothecarists) were perceived as having achieved mixed successes, with some discoveries offering good results and some ending up with results that had exceedingly bad outcomes. Some societies viewed them as supplying hope for cures, other viewed them as witches and medieval potion makers. It is sufficient to say most early scientists really did not have a clue what was going on and why certain treatments worked. The risk-to-benefit safety discussions would not evolve as being essential to treatment plans for many centuries.

The earliest medical doctors recommended crude treatments like bloodletting and drainage of pus, isolation, quarantine, and natural responses like sweating the infection away as natural observed God-given mechanisms to address illness. It took thousands of years to understand how the immune system functioned, and it is still a bit of a mystery often left to experts who claim to know more than other citizens, even without understood science to support their claims. A commonsense approach would demand science be understood and explained, but the adage if it happens somewhere, then there must be science to explain the natural occurrence most certainly applies to reported observations.

As it turns out, the human body has a powerful immune system, which forms a natural protection on its own and can adapt to infectious diseases and fight off infection, also known as natural immunity which serves as the basis for curing illness for ages. Some plants and herbs acting as drugs helped, and some aggressive therapies also seemed to help even if it simply meant resting and allowing the immune system and other protective systems to establish a natural balance, like prompting a fever to fight off the infection. Noble Liars and servants of elites remained liars because no one had the science to call them out as liars. Science would become stagnant for centuries along with the pursuit of better lives for individuals.

However, it was often a wild time as entire royal (ruling) families died, and many poor families rose in status as someone had to lead society, as again infectious diseases are not discriminatory. False science and leaders scrambled in historical outbreaks which also applies to leaders during infectious outbreaks today. To address such false science, citizens must demand facts and discoveries be addressed through scientific methodology and the science must be universally recorded and available to all citizens. Where today oddly many companies provide internet resources to help citizens, yet our government looks to limit and hide access to science to limited groups of authorities with higher discretionary powers.

Science often takes centuries to learn and understand. Which as related to infectious disease discoveries, Robert Hooke is credited with describing the fruiting structures of molds in 1665 and Antoni van Leeuwenhoek is recognized with the discovery of bacteria in 1676. The first virus discovered was not until 1892 and that was a tobacco mosaic virus, followed by a foot-and-mouth disease virus in 1898. The first human virus was the yellow fever virus in 1901. New species of human viruses are still being found at a rate of about three or four per year. Viruses make up over two-thirds of all known and new human infectious pathogens (or "germs") when combined with bacteria, fungi, and helminths (parasitic worms) as the common human pathogens.

Several key areas of treatment have been discovered and developed in the last century covering a wide range of pathogens. Viruses being the simplest of the two common infectious pathogens. Bacterium being the other primary leading cause of infectious disease. Viruses are the smallest pathogen and the quickest to adapt to change, making it often the hardest to treat effectively. Strands of virus can undergo genetic replication and adaption far faster than the human body can adapt to the change in the body's environment and produce an immune defense. Bacteria are slower to change; rather than being strands of genetic material, they are comprised of infectious cells which are far more complex, but far less likely to change or adapt to a treatment.

Viruses are faster and nimbler, and scientists have not figured out how to completely shut down the replication process without also causing other adverse drug responses. Bacterial infections on the other hand have been understood and widely addressed using antibiotic therapies. Pharmaceutical science can explain many of the adverse side effects and complications antibiotics cause today. Yet, antibiotics are becoming less effective, as the complex cell structure of bacteria can adapt over time and make antibiotics less effective, which is often referred to as antibiotic resistance, so the antibiotic starts to fail as a treatment option, usually requiring a switch to one or many other types of antibiotics or drug protocols. There are many classes of antibiotics, each with differing antibacterial actions and uses among numerous bacterial infections.

As competing pathogens, bacterial infections are now manageable by historical standards, but viruses continue to be a less successfully controlled infectious disease. Other pathogens like worms and funguses are also complex parasites inside the body and often have poor or limited treatment protocols. Treatment protocols have improved but can be difficult to treat if not administered in the early stages of the infectious disease.

Before the 19th century, scientists had a trivial understanding of a complex immune system. Immunity was often considered a gift of God or something one was born with, like being from a good family. Those ideas still exist today, as many scientists point to genetics and the gift of good health from acquired immunity and good hygiene practices taught and passed down through the family and social setting. For centuries, it was not fully known that mothers often passed along immune antibodies through the placenta before birth and with breastfeeding, which gives their babies passive immunity to many diseases. And passive immunity can be passed from one family member to other family members or close relations, but the level of passive immunity is often insufficient to be effective against all infectious diseases, as the level of antibodies developed by passive immunity may be marginal or limited by other factors.

These ideas of natural and passive immunity have existed for centuries. A healthy and strong immune system is a combination of many things and a bit of luck, along with good nutrition and other healthy body systems. Among the earliest recorded scientists to provoke immunity in humans were farmers and doctors who used a practice called variolation (or inoculation), which was a discovery made that an infection can be controlled in an animal and humans with a less lethal natural form of smallpox called Variola Minor. If exposed to Variola Minor, the animals and humans would be protected from reinfection when later exposed to the more lethal form of infection called Variola Major. This practice of variolation had been used since ancient times in India and China long before the practice was introduced to Europe in the 1700s. Variolation had a distinct disadvantage in that the antigen (agent) used still contained an active form of smallpox, which was less potent and less infectious than Variola Major but could still kill the immunized person or spread the infectious disease to others. The death rates of Variola Minor were just 2% as compared to a death rate of almost 20% or more in the more serious Variola Major patients. This was the earliest version of using the development of similar antibody types to develop protective immunity as an observed tradeoff of using similar antigens to lessen the more complicated infectious disease outcomes. Getting sick with one infectious disease, Variola Minor, gave protection from a more serious infectious disease, Variola Major. This was an acceptable option to many citizens during the Middle Ages. It was not an absolute positive tradeoff in fully addressing the illness, but variolation was an observed scientific fact-based tradeoff observed over many centuries and considered an acceptable tradeoff by many citizens, especially farmers interested in protecting their livestock animals.

The first vaccine was discovered in 1796, by Dr. Edward Jenner, a rural British doctor who had practiced variolation and had heard about a tradition of using cowpox (from cows) to confer immunity to smallpox, as the cowpox was much less fatal to humans. Originally demonstrated as a method for immunization by Benjamin Jesty, a farmer, Dr. Jenner extended Jesty's observations and documented how cowpox could be passed from lesions of handmaids to others through forearm to forearm transfers. The last person with a lesion and exposed to cowpox was also found to be immune to smallpox. Cowpox being a far much less deadly disease than smallpox. Dr. Jenner described the procedure and documented his results, then distributed his vaccine discovery freely to others. The smallpox vaccine within decades became a widely used method to induce protection as it became the primary drug used by many European and American physicians in the treatment of smallpox. Interestingly, Dr. Jenner was an empiricist, who believed science discoveries come from observed or sensed empirical scientific evidence. During the Middle Ages, empiricism evolved into the fundamental requirement for applying scientific methods to test all hypothesis and theories against observations noted or found in nature. Empiricists used *a posteriori* logic or Latin for "from the latter" to refer to a form of logic that works from the discovered effects backwards to its cause, as developed from science methods of documenting knowledge learned from a scientist's observations. Which is different from *a priori* knowledge, which involves logic in making conclusions and arguments that exist independent of one's experience of observed facts and relates to knowledge or reasoning that comes from some theoretical assumption about nature.

I mention this here, as I find it interesting vaccine discoveries started under the logic of scientists who practiced the *a posteriori* empirical method of science. Yet today some vaccine scientists and lawyers have evolved into experts that practice *a priori* scientific logic in explaining science in vaccine courts, as I will explain later in the book. Lawyers demand the empirical evidence and facts, for cause and effect relationship and making decisions; but generally use their instincts and assumption of nature to fill in gaps and often make flawed opinions about science and scientific relationships. Two different approaches to science and logic, *a priori* formed independent of observed experiences or knowledge, while a *posteriori* uses logic for knowledge formed based on observation and learned experiences. Our current vaccine laws and the original vaccine discoveries are based on two different lines of logic and knowledge. A difference between law and medicine that has separated the two professions for centuries, yet now dramatically changes how science is understood and applied to vaccines in a court of law. The laws of nature observed by scientists are gradually slipping to science credited to experts who have not observed the science but speculate and postulate on what the expected science should be. Judges do not base evidence on *a posteriori* empiric evidence, but on speculative statements of evidence which are open to misinterpretation and misunderstanding.

But back to Dr. Jenner who published his findings and advanced the first vaccine to be used for the widely scourged infectious disease smallpox. The theories to support further advances in vaccines however did not evolve for almost another century. The observation and recorded discovery of a vaccine was made by Dr. Jenner and others that followed his procedures in making similar vaccines, but scientists and doctors did not understand the immune system or how such protective immunity was formed in the body based upon his findings or observations. Empirical evidence showing that vaccines were evidently and repeatedly used to control smallpox outbreaks without much noted adverse injuries was good enough at the time. Vaccines were considered a miracle drug, or magic at the time.

The understanding that vaccines created the same immune response as infectious diseases, without all the major complications of the disease, and a patient would develop protection without having the full-blown infection, provided a clearer path to understanding an inner complexity to our body systems which was not fully documented by scientists as an inner-body process prior to Dr. Jenner's observation. This newer understanding provided a path to treatments for many infections, or at least the very worst infectious diseases, it was hoped. Today, smallpox is generally considered eradicated and is used as a promotional tool to advocate hope that other vaccines will one day lead to eradication of other infectious diseases. A nice promotional thought to offer to the public, but completely misses some of the science which nonscientists often overlook relating to poorly understood adverse reactions and vaccine safety concerns.

The U.S. government began its first official promotional campaign for a vaccine in 1813 (17 years after Dr. Jenner's discovery in England), when Congress authorized and President James Madison signed an Act into law that encouraged all American citizens should be vaccinated and established the young nation's first National Vaccine Agency, with James Smith, a physician, being appointed as the first National Vaccine Agent. The United States Postal Service at the time was required to carry all mail weighing up to 0.5 ounces for free if the packaged mailed contained any material part of the smallpox vaccine. These actions demonstrated the U.S. government's dedication to fund and promote a discovery that was still in its infancy, giving our government a meaningful tie to vaccines many in our government still feel obligated to preserving today as a protected bond, worthy of protecting at all costs. And the vaccine promotional efforts serve as proof that even as two nations (England and the newly formed United States of America) can be enemies, as the War of 1812 was only a year earlier, important science can be understood in all nations regardless of politics and national interests. Which oddly today, some American-based scientists (doctors) and nonscientists (like VICP special masters) think the only pure and validated science is introduced and discovered in the United States, and that American doctors are in some way the "greatest doctors and scientists in the world".

As science progressed, in the latter half of the 1800s, Louis Pasteur of France disproved and rejected the popular theory, at the time, of spontaneous generation. The earlier scientific idea that living matter could spontaneously be created from nonliving matter, which led him to devise the modern theory of infectious disease, suggesting specific microorganisms cause specific diseases, and he then proceeded to isolate the infectious disease anthrax and altered the infectious bacteria. He then introduced the inactivated bacterium into farm animals, which he then proved induced immunity to the disease without the deadly effects of the disease. Pasteur also isolated rabies using a similar inactivation process of preparing a vaccine for rabies. Not that these early vaccines did not cause problems or serious adverse effects, they did, but the newly discovered methodology suggestively solved a serious infectious disease concern using a new path to creating additional vaccines.

However, scientists still did not understand how the complete immune system worked and the lack in understand the presence of antibodies (also called immunoglobulins), and a fully developed immune and lymphatic system until the late nineteenth century and early twentieth century. Emil von Behring and Shibasabura Kitasato published in 1890 a study that showed the transfer of serum from animals immunized against diphtheria to animals suffering from the disease could effectively "cure" the infected animals by a process suggested as a transfer of a substance thought to be what they called "antibodies".

On the human side, several vaccines were developed in the late 1800s and early 1900s including antitoxins against diphtheria, tetanus, anthrax, cholera, plague, typhoid, tuberculosis, and other vaccines were developed. Several of the vaccines were modestly successful, at the time proclaiming to be breakthroughs as there were no effective treatments for these infectious diseases. The noted adverse events related to the vaccines were still a major concern but far better than the alternative of having no drug available to treat these terrible infectious diseases. This firmly establishing the earliest claims that a vaccine offered protective benefits that are far more important than any suggested adverse side effects from the vaccine. Adverse vaccine-related events at first thought to be related to the illness itself and not the vaccine, where it was thought the vaccine was administered just in time before the disease kicked in, so the vaccines were thought of as being both protective and a treatment. The understanding that vaccines mimic an infectious disease and can independently cause adverse reactions was not yet fully understood. Most suspected adverse reactions of vaccines were considered far less serious than the complications of the infectious disease, which became the early vaccine promotional mantra, which is still used today. Or in caveman-terms: vaccine good, infections bad, adverse reactions who cares, became the standard argument for vaccine use.

This is not to say any of these infectious diseases disappeared or were eradicated from societies. The human vaccine experiment simply kicked into a higher gear. Many classes of drugs became experimental agents tested and tried on many citizens. Many individuals were poor or had few healthcare options other than a limited number of public hospitals, public health clinics, and a few community doctors and community pharmacies. Experimental practices and promotion of medical treatment options sometimes harmed patients, and sometimes led to discoveries, and in the vaccine-class of drugs allowed several vaccines to establish safer dosing and vaccine manufacturing processes. Vaccines also served as a tool for spreading democracy and capitalism as being the best economic model for other countries of the world to embrace. Vaccines were an early path to cheap and mostly effective protection against diseases as the government sought expansion through commercial development and projects in other nations, and these new territories often required addressing a serious infectious disease. A lot like China has adopted its current policy for expanding its influence across many nations and seeking to conquer many infectious diseases often with antibiotics and less expensive pharmaceuticals, but still not entirely addressing the vaccine safety issue. Although China has made more efforts to address vaccine-related injuries in recent years.

In this period from the late 1800s to early 1900s, other vaccine developments included vaccines that were developed for what was determined to be diseases caused by toxins that are released by bacteria rather than a disease caused by the bacteria itself. Tetanus is an example of a bacteria that often killed a person much faster than the time it took the immune system to recognize the toxin and produce antibodies against the toxin. The tetanus toxin was denatured, using the process of creating a vaccine known as a toxoid. These vaccines created antibodies to protect against the bacterium, which in turn protected the body against the toxins. Very smart science and novel, but again did not address vaccine safety issues, although some of these methods were considered as safer and more specific to the cause and not activating as many adverse effects. At least not adverse events any scientists were monitoring at the time.

The typhoid vaccine is also interesting, as it was developed to treat what was originally thought to be a virus. Typhus and typhoid fever are actually two separate diseases caused by two different bacteria (not viruses), with similar names but different bacterial causes and was often confused as being related in some way when first discovered. A vaccine was developed for typhoid fever, but today is not generally needed as it is a bacterium treatable with antibiotics. Back in 1906, a story circulated in the New York newspaper media of a ship cook, nicknamed by the journalists as Typhoid Mary, who came over on a ship and passed typhoid fever to 53 fellow travelers (3 who died), unaware that she was an asymptomatic carrier of typhoid fever disease. The story serves as a popular reference and is a passed down as a story of why many citizens and authorities consider all vaccines vital to our safety for protection against any infectious disease, especially those with a risk of asymptomatic spread of the disease. A bit of nonsensical logic as the times and treatment plans have changed as both typhus and typhoid fever are treated with antibiotics making a vaccine unnecessary for most areas where the disease once prevailed.

In the same period, the U.S. Supreme Court in 1905 heard the case of *Jacobson v. Massachusetts* and upheld the constitutionality of mandatory smallpox vaccination programs as a method of preserving public health, a policy the Supreme Court still upholds today, as implied public health is considered of being higher in importance than public safety and protection from vaccine-related injuries. The media image of a Typhoid Mary in every infectious outbreak and the Supreme Court's 1905 decision serve as popular legal references of why legal professionals are taught vaccines are vital to public health, and endorse the idea that vaccine safety will never be addressed by the Court. Not that vaccine laws have changed for the worse regarding vaccine safety and promotion, they did improve but have since taken a major step back since 1986. Our government has failed to change with the times and still holds to its roots of promoting vaccine use and overlooking vaccine safety concerns. A sort of one step forward, two step backwards sort of problem for vaccine safety concerns and how they should be addressed by medical professionals and our government.

Other vaccines discovered in this timeframe included Cholera, which is also a bacterium-related infectious disease, which would later be treated with antibiotics and other therapeutic protocols. And plague, including Black Plague, continued as a long-standing infectious concern but was never understood to be caused by a bacterium until the 1980s. In fact, a lot of other discoveries were made while trying to find vaccines for plague and influenza infectious diseases. Cholera vaccines are still around today but are not considered necessary in most countries with good sanitary systems, as the vaccine was largely thought to protect against bacterial infections no one understood at the time. The original purpose for these vaccines were noble ideas, but the development of antibiotics and other drugs and improved healthier living conditions led to better options for controlling these infectious diseases.

In this period, the promotional idea of wiping away disease with vaccines also became actively promoted. In the first half of the 1900s, Tuberculosis, Pertussis, Diphtheria, Yellow fever, Influenza, Tetanus toxoid, and Rickettsia vaccines were all developed. Again, these vaccines all had mixed results and sometimes serious adverse side effects. A major infectious outbreak, the Spanish flu outbreak in 1918 changed research on infectious diseases a lot. The cause of the Spanish flu was a virus, an H1N1 type influenza virus, similar but not identical to the 2009 H1N1 outbreak. The viral outbreak occurred in a pre-antibiotic era, and there were no therapeutic treatments to effectively treat secondary infections. The spread and impact of the Spanish flu virus was profoundly serious, as the highly contagious virus was widespread and serious. An estimated 100 million people died from the Spanish flu outbreak (equivalent to approximately 5% of the world's population at the time). No pandemic, epidemic or plague since has even come close to the widespread complications of the Spanish flu. Yet every new or novel viral outbreak since has been compared to or designated as being the next Spanish flu-like pandemic. Again, the Spanish flu was a pre-antibiotic era infectious outbreak. COVID and other influenza outbreaks have been compared to the Spanish flu, but again are not even close as real-life medical concerns, as it was a different time and different set of therapeutic treatment options available today versus 1918.

Vaccines had a good, century-long run of the infectious disease research and development science until in 1928 Alexander Fleming discovered penicillin, ironically an accidental discovery as he was doing research for an influenza vaccine. The discovery of antibiotics one could say was the start of a new era in infectious disease drug history, as penicillin became a widely used drug for many infectious diseases. Other antibiotics followed including tetracycline and erythromycin, and others. Research and development of antibiotics exploded, and more favorable routes of administration were developed. Antibiotics easily surpassed vaccines as a preferred treatment option for many infectious diseases that were bacterial-based infections. Not all infectious diseases, like virus-based infections, were covered by antibiotics, as researchers discovered antibiotics had no benefit in fighting viral-based infections but did serve to treat complicated secondary bacterial infections. More research and better tools like bacterial type testing and higher quality microscopes were developed in the first decades of the 1900s, bacteria cell structures first being discovered in the late 1800s and viral structures a couple of decades later, which made matching therapeutic antibiotics and treating bacterial infections more easily available and determining the proper treatment protocols for specific diseases. Viruses remained a dilemma, and vaccines remained the sole drug of choice for viral-based infectious diseases until the 1980s.

The antibiotics developed were superior therapeutic treatments for bacterial infections. Vaccines only offered hope for desired protection against bacterial infectious diseases through antibody development. In time, the distinction between protective and therapeutic treatments became clearer to doctors and scientists. Vaccines continued to be developed but fell somewhat out of favor, as patients preferred to wait and see if an infectious disease developed and if there was an absolute need for protective treatments, giving favor to natural antibody development, and to avoid some of the problematic side effects of vaccines, including the general feeling of going through an illness-like medical complication that often made the vaccinated patient feel extremely sick, with adverse symptoms that were not set apart as concerns and few scientists made efforts to document the adverse reactionary events considered to be vaccine-related.

The history of adverse drug reactions or events (also called ADRs or ADEs) picked up as a concern in this timeframe following the wider public concerns for many drugs. An ADR is defined as an injury caused by a drug, alone or in combination with other drugs or related to injuries caused by and relating to certain medical mechanisms of action. The study of ADRs is known as pharmacovigilance, and an adverse drug event refers to any injury occurring in the same timeframe as a drug is being used to treat a patient. These adverse events are important regardless of whether or not the drug is identified as the sole or combined source for a related cause of a drug-induced injury. An ADR is marked as being related to the drug being administered until proven as unrelated or understood through scientific research. An ADR is often demonstrated to have a causative relationship that in fact led to a drug-related injury, or can be related to missing or not taking a drug for a medical condition, as therapy may be inaccurately dosed or related to drug metabolism issues. Too bad most lawyers do not understand ADRs, as that could help them understand more vaccine safety and drug adverse reaction issues. Most lawyers still living in the theoretical world of theoretical (not real or observed science) causational logic for cause and effect determinations, as they form their beliefs on what they expect to be the cause and effect and not necessarily what is observed through empirical evidence. In medicine and pharmacy, an ADR is an ADR until proven to be caused by something else, which in the case of vaccines today is often overlooked or discounted as being caused or are assigned by authorities to be due to something else, even as doctors rarely have a fully understood explanation for the vaccine-related ADR.

Adverse drug reactions began to be evaluated more carefully in the 1930's and led to the enactment of the Food Drug and Cosmetics Act. In this Act, ADRs were classified in relationship to causation and severity and into two types of reactions: Type A pharmacological effects which were generally dose dependent and predictable and initially thought to represent almost 80% of all ADRs, and Type B pharmacological ADRs which were labelled idiosyncratic, meaning no one really knows what was causing the ADR. Perhaps a type B ADR was possibly related to the drug's mechanisms of action or dosing, or individual concerns such as children and elderly often had widely differing responses to many drugs related to body systems. As pharmacovigilance science improved in the 1960s and 1970s, additional types of adverse drug reactions were proposed, added, and researched as the simple two type (A and B) labelling system proved a failure to classify many ADRs. True pharmacovigilance reporting and analysis started in this period.

These failures to understand ADRs included many serious drug reactions. Vaccines were part of this wide group of drugs with poorly understood adverse drug reactions, and vaccine safety concerns quickly became a widely recognized concern among citizens deciding which drugs worked and which were unsafe. In the United States, the FDA defines the seriousness of an ADR as possible outcomes including death, resulting in a life-threatening complication, causing hospitalization (at onset of taking a drug or after a prolonged time of being on a drug), disability (in many forms of both short and long-term disability), causing congenital defects, or requiring an intervention to prevent permanent impairment or damage. These concerns are mostly based on an arbitrary scale of seriousness, often using an arbitrary judgement made by both patients and clinicians in determining whether the ADR is severe, serious, or rated down to minor or rare. The broad terms are often used interchangeably and can often be misapplied or confused even by trained professionals. For example, simple judgements of a severe headache often using a scale of 1 to 10. This may help explain the pain level, but does nothing to address the seriousness of the headache which could be due to increased levels of inflammation or as serious as a brain cerebrovascular event which can be due to many causes and may be related to many drugs.

I will state here that vaccines have a poor history of pharmacovigilance reporting which fail the standard ADR typing test, as many adverse vaccine reactions are deemed idiopathic or unknown, until a few scientists began to understand or research the concerns in the 1970s. Many adverse vaccine safety concerns were shelved in early vaccines as being complex idiopathic medical concerns. However, in 1976, a group of doctors investigated an adverse vaccine reaction related to the Swine flu vaccine and concluded it was the cause of Guillain-Barre Syndrome (also called GBS). The doctors investigating the cause of GBS, including Maurice Hilleman, Joseph Bellanti (my vaccine injury case expert) and other scientists, addressed the adverse vaccine response at Fort Dix in New Jersey, and determined the cause of the adverse event was linked to the Swine flu vaccine, and that the vaccine-related injury must be addressed without delay even as the rate of occurrence was considered rare.

Merck, the high-flying Swine flu's vaccine manufacturer, had aggressively agreed to produce up to 50 million Swine flu vaccine doses in January 1977 and had delivered almost 11 million doses in late January 1976, an aggressive position authorized by Congress as our government authorities were committed to vaccine funding to address the suspected serious Swine flu outbreak. Not much different than the current aggressive actions taken to pay out multiple manufacturers for hundreds of millions of COVID vaccine doses. In 1976, the nationwide Swine flu vaccine program ended promptly after vaccinations were associated to increased risks of GBS. GBS has many causes including a bacterial infection from the bacteria called *Campylobacter,* but recipients of the Swine flu vaccine experienced a higher than normal rate of occurrence than the general population of about 1 additional case per 100,000 vaccine recipients. And despite what many scientists and the government promised to be a widespread outbreak of Swine flu, only a few cases of the actual infectious disease ever developed among American citizens.

In this widely observed VACCINE fiasco, the FDA and government intervened, even as the "seriousness" of the GBS vaccine injury was deemed less complicated and arbitrarily assigned as a minor concern even as the vaccine injury could cause long-term and permanent neurological damage. The level of seriousness was uncertain as to what extent the adverse drug reaction caused long-term damage, but vaccine manufacturers immediately feared the worst, and threatened to pull out of the U.S. vaccine market unless the government intervened. The government obliged with experts from the FDA and interestingly the Department of Justice offering lawyers to help craft a solution. The doctors and government lawyers of course did not come to an agreement, but the lawyers won out in helping "save" the vaccine manufacturers whom the DOJ feared would end vaccine distribution for lack of profit and higher development costs, often relating to rising legal liability costs. Most outside parties today would call it a government bailout, a bailout of a long ongoing partnership with a vaccine promotional program that had been going on for over 150 years.

Most citizens do not realize vaccines almost reached a level of being restricted or obsolete in the U.S. and in other countries in the 1970s and 1980s. Yes, vaccines were still available and promoted but many citizens were refusing them based on ADRs, and reflected little effort by the FDA to address vaccine ADRs, which often went undocumented or addressed in pharmacovigilance reporting. The ADR problem related to egg allergies was understood, but most adverse vaccine drug reactions were simply dismissed as undocumented, listed as marginal in rate of frequency, and having undetermined causation, or were idiopathic and thought to be easily addressed with standard treatment protocols. The need to isolate and address vaccine ADRs was minimalized and dismissed until the 1976 Swine Flu fiasco hit the public and created a media panic.

At this point in drug history, antibiotics had a substantial lead as the bacterial drug treatment of choice, and antibiotics had well-developed safety profiles where doctors could quickly identify and address the cause and seriousness of an ADR. Most doctors fully understood the safety profiles of various antibiotics, and pharmacovigilance reporting for antibiotics was better than reporting for many drug classes, which was considered as a fair balance of safety versus benefits for the many antibiotics being manufactured. Vaccines had less-understood adverse safety records, but the protective actions of vaccines were known and thought to be good protective treatments if matched right. Vaccine promotion by our government still held out hope for eradication as a desired outcome if promotion were continued, but the cost to make and research vaccines continued to skyrocket in relationship to sales. Vaccine manufacturers feared new and more deeply researched adverse vaccine injuries would conflict with continued research and development, and certainly make it more difficult to make a profit. During this period, vaccine research by pharmaceutical manufacturers began to lose favor, even as more immune system science and mechanisms of vaccine and immune system actions continued to be discovered, with suggestive therapeutic uses for vaccines as possibly being used as therapeutic drugs to treat a wide range of medical conditions.

While vaccines lost market share to antibiotics, a newer drug class also began to be researched since antibiotics did not cover viral infections, only working as a treatment for bacterial infections. The newer class of drugs were antiviral drugs, which were designed to treat viral infections therapeutically rather than providing suggestive protection against viral diseases. The mechanisms of action for antivirals were scientifically proven, but the development of effective antivirals took a little longer to research and develop. Vaccines, however, were on the way out for many researchers and manufacturers, as the problems and safety were highly uncertain, the costs to develop a vaccine was slow and costly, and acceptance by the public was becoming marginal. And the overhead costs relating to legal liability were a huge growing concern.

The government stepping in and addressing these liability concerns changed everything, even as many doctors and other pharmaceutical parties did not agree with the action of granting vaccines exclusive protection which was unheard of for any drug class. The government's legal intervention and protection of vaccines was not only unfair for competitive reasons, but unfair as it does not address the safety concerns in a fair and ongoing manner, meaning citizens could be financially harmed as our government can fail to address the vaccine ADR concerns with little recourse or protection of a citizen's legal right to seek damage from a vaccine injury.

The government made numerous claims and promises to win concessions in Congress and "agreed" to address vaccine safety concerns in-house through the VICP and FDA, suggesting the FDA, CDC, and other research parties could effectively manage and address the concerns. However, all parties, including vaccine manufacturers, have since failed to properly address vaccine safety concerns. Vaccine manufacturers changed the vaccine reporting process for ADRs, with variable and different reporting in different countries and some vaccine safety concerns being shelved for extended periods. This was not a good thing for the citizens as the ongoing vaccine safety issues would not be addressed in a fair and rapid manner. Some countries quickly opted out of this scheme and began their own vaccine regulatory and safety programs and agencies. And even as our government promised to address vaccine safety issues in some fair manner, the task became much harder than had originally been anticipated and in 1995 the Department of Health and Human Services shifted strategies and created a Vaccine Injury Table to separate claims into different classifications and levels of proof for causation and sequential timing relating to a vaccine injury claim. This action was taken with limited medical community input, shifting the burden on claims to be limiting and focusing on well-defined injuries related to each vaccine that have understood or well-defined relationships relating to timing and defined causation.

Therefore, certain vaccine-injury claims would be paid in a more automatic fashion. The idea being, at least for lawyers, if the cause and timing were understood, a simple process of paying out the settlement of a vaccine-injury claim would be simplified for all parties and the costs would be reduced and paid out more efficiently. What more could any citizen expect from government officials other than taking actions that would cut costs and make the program suggestively more efficient, at least easier for the lawyers? However, this action alone changed the Vaccine Act's legislated promise, as the government edged forward at a crawl with vaccine-related concerns not included in the Vaccine Table. These understood ADRs and concerns are still debated today. Efforts to make changes and additions to the Vaccine Table are unbearably slow, and the DOJ aggressively litigates every off-Table Vaccine Injury, as the injuries are suggested not to be vaccine-related, even as more recent studies and science shows that many of the injuries are related to the administered vaccines. Some vaccines are exceptionally poorly addressed such as the influenza vaccine which changes formulations every year. Doctors called before the VICP court would often make statements of uncertainty as many doctors are not vaccine experts and often could not fully see the causal relationship and mechanisms of injury, as they had not studied or observed the adverse events in their practices.

Going back to discoveries, Immunologists Dr. Jonas Salk, Dr. Albert Sabin (Abram Saperstejn), Dr. Joseph Bellanti and other colleagues made key discoveries that would open vaccines to another era of protective and therapeutic treatments. These discoveries were promising, and even groundbreaking, but adverse drug reaction problems persisted. For example, in 1955 the U.S. Surgeon General suspended the recently developed polio vaccination program to investigate the safety of all six polio vaccine manufacturers. The review of eleven deaths and hundreds of immunized patients becoming paralyzed was thought to be conclusive, but never officially proven or accepted. The government later suggested the cause was related to a production method error failing to completely kill the Type 1 poliovirus as instructed by Dr. Salk, the scientist who discovered the vaccine.

The vaccines as a drug class again were costly to discover, somewhat inexpensive to manufacture, but had highly fluctuating costs especially for certain types of vaccines, and were costly to market to the public, and unfortunately were developing a higher liability cost, as many viral vaccines were found to have adverse risks not previously disclosed. In the 1976 Swine flu fiasco, the implied added incidence for risk of GBS was small (0.001%), and the government pushed the narrative that vaccines as a class of drugs with "unknown" ADRs are largely considered safe and effective. And, as legislated and adopted in the Vaccine Act in 1986, independent of any science, vaccines became mostly liability-free and openly promoted as safe and effective drugs, with only a few cases of rare ADRs following a vaccine administration infrequently being listed as adverse concerns.

The government happily promoted good fortune for all vaccines, even as some vaccines like influenza vaccines had effectiveness rates that only rarely went over a rate of being more than 50% effective, and in fact, in many years fell below 10% effectiveness. Just think, would any citizen take a drug with a sketchy drug-related safety profile and only a 10% chance the drug would work, for say, a heart condition? An antibiotic with such a profile would instantly be rejected in the drug marketplace. Yet the government stuck with the vaccines, especially viral vaccines, which in the 1980s had few alternatives. And just to be clear, there are numerous viruses that cause from mild to severe infectious complications. As noted, prior to antibiotics this was a serious problem, as the viral infection creates a favorable environment for bacterial infections to jump and take off, so even if the viral infection may be manageable, when in combination with secondary bacterial infections it can become difficult to manage.

Yet, new antibiotics made it possible to effectively manage most bacterial infections, and often the viral infection became a less complicated infection to treat. Often doctors just do not know which protocol to choose in managing such concerns, and the patient becomes more ill from the secondary infection, not the viral infection which was labelled as being the primary infection. Such poor judgements have become less frequent as treatment plans and testing for bacterial types have greatly improved in recent decades. But testing often occurs in a clinical hospital setting and can take days, which again is improving but has a lot of room for improvement. A day or two of an aggressive viral infection can make a big difference, in how the infection may be manifested and treated and outcomes related to the treatment plan.

After 1986, the U.S. government officially "silently" changed from being a vaccine drug regulator, to actively being a vaccine promotor, a vaccine drug litigation resolution program, and a selective drug regulator often acting as a selective watchdog with selective oversight often directed by political interests and self-interests, as well as political lobbyists interested in critical decisions that impacted their financial profitability. Between 1976 and 1986, vaccine research and development investments were slowing down considerably. However, medical researchers were also discovering new vaccine mechanisms of action, down to the cell function, which at the time was revolutionary. Today, scientists are down to the intracellular protein function, and intercellular cross talk mechanisms in research. Vaccine pharmaceutical chemistry and mechanisms of action research opened new options for research and development and new suggestive uses for new therapeutic disease treatment options. Forget vaccine protective mechanisms many companies thought of as the sole reason for administering vaccines. The future would be in therapeutic uses of vaccines for cancer and other diseases. A vaccine liability protection would buffer against required vaccine safety creating the supreme business wild card in the field of vaccine and pharmaceutical research and development.

After the Vaccine Act was enacted in 1986, vaccine manufacturers had the coveted golden ticket, and it was time to open the vaccine research and development flood gate. The vaccine business was officially back "in business" as they say. Vaccine manufacturers like Merck and Sanofi and others jumped right in, with new research and a return of some older vaccines with new twists. The resulting research for some new vaccines were sketchy, as the vaccine science became more closely guarded, you know for proprietary (commercial) reasons of course. The science also expanded to focus on more vaccinations needing to be administered to children, which is interesting as limited prospective studies had never been approved to evaluate adverse injuries to many vaccines noted in children. Such a prospective study would be labelled unethical to test a child under the age of 18, regardless of a parent's consent. The area of law surrounding medical choice and regulation was thrown into a cyclone of poor judgements in the decades that followed the Vaccine Act, but vaccine research and development was definitively back.

Pharmaceutical companies, both those in the vaccine business and those with interest in the actions of vaccines, perked up, and over the next few decades, from 1986 to today, vaccines have become the "it" drug class for pharmaceutical research and development teams. And government promotional teams and research funding programs could not be happier. The push to eradicate many diseases globally accelerated but did not include an increase in safety and adverse risk evaluation teams, leaving vaccine manufacturers to explore new territories, as the government has granted the manufacturers and medical professionals immunity to virtually all legal liability. What does any party have to lose? The idea of exploration and funding new science spread, and much of the research became funded under the government's National Institutes of Health (or NIH) grants and partnerships.

The government had stated they would be extremely cautious in addressing any safety concerns when legislating the Vaccine Act, but the government clearly did not intervene to address vaccine safety concerns when adverse events became observed and reported. Rather, they acted as an intermediary to pharmaceutical manufacturers' interests. The regulatory vaccine concerns mandated by regulatory agencies, like the FDA, slipped as public and certainly medical professional interest in vaccine safety declined, and the interest of supporting "new" vaccine science and uses moved forward. This interest did not only affect vaccines, but greatly impacted many new classes of drugs that the FDA granted wider protections to under a broader regulatory umbrella. Old drugs, like PPA, ephedrine, and quinine were out, as their safety risks are documented and were known from decades of evidence to have serious ADRs; and drugs like biological and newer classes of cutting edge drugs, including vaccines are in, despite limited and poorly developed safety profiles. Some drug approvals seemingly approved by the FDA simply to give the manufacturer time to recoup their research and investment costs, as a drug's patent expires way too fast for some parties with a window to recoup costs falling to less than 10 years in the case of many FDA approved drugs. Our government and the FDA has pushed to be recognized as world leaders in medical and drug innovation, where drug safety has fallen down the ladder as an issue that must be addressed to be considered a healthcare leader to some parties.

The United States government, effective 1986, was officially in the drug business, the vaccine drug business to be specific, which was something many citizens already knew, as pharmaceutical drug lobbyists have long played a role in Washington, D.C.. But now, the government was officially in the protection business, for commercial interests, and it was their duty to strengthen their alliance. Do citizens understand this? Probably not. Just as citizens did not understand the dangers of controlled substances in the 1950s and earlier, where amphetamines were sold over-the-counter in pharmacies as alertness pills and opiates were long used for pain and other medicinal purposes going back centuries. Citizens are not at the outset generally informed or educated to adverse drug risks. Our government historically fails in the drug safety department. Always has and likely always will. Citizens can change that and demand safety first, which would be a step in the right direction.

A discussion on drug history stretches into another conversation on drug laws and drug law enforcement. Another subject for another time perhaps, as many drug laws are poorly supported by science and facts understood and researched by scientists. Are some drug laws outdated and given too much discretion allowing too few authorities to decide what is best for citizens? Now is as good of a time as any to demand changes in some of our drug laws and the need to shift resources to providing citizen education and tools to help citizens in making better and informed healthcare choices.

After the 1986 Vaccine Act, new vaccine discoveries exploded with an average of one to three new vaccines being researched every year. Many are now in clinical trials for novel treatment options for medical conditions like cancers, dental caries (cavities), hookworms, Alzheimer's, and more. Citizens must understand when you sign up for a clinical trial, you are often giving away your rights to sue for adverse side effects and damages caused to your body by any novel therapeutic treatments. In the case of vaccines, the liability for research and development and manufacturing falls to almost zero. But do not be concerned that you may be a human lab test subject, one step above a lab animal, as most clinical trials are now done overseas, in countries with large populations, like China, but not so much in India, where many citizens are very well educated and protective of their culture, and they offer no patent protections for almost anything.

The days of human experimentation with vaccines as a suggestive drug tool have been opened up again for not just American citizens but for citizens around the world, and it is not an arms race but a wide-open vaccine drug race to see who can lead the world and perhaps find novel and safe vaccines for many uses including infectious diseases and other therapeutic uses. China, India, and other countries are not just in the cheap drug business, they are in the global pharmaceutical cutting-edge drug business. And if they can make vaccines safer, a doubtful proposition, they could also lead the way to a wider selection of vaccines. A noble goal for citizens, but likely a waste of money and valuable resources which could be used in other healthcare programs and drug therapies.

If a citizen is in a vaccine clinical trial, the citizen should understand the risks of ADRs (adverse drug reactions) are not clearly defined but can be profoundly serious and complicated. Some risks are still not fully understood and rather than researching the risks further, a patient that is found to have an ADR in a clinical study is promptly removed from the study. This does not further any understanding of the risk, but simply removes the patient from the likely list of adverse risks caused by the vaccine, where doctors will try other drugs to find some balance and return body systems back to normal. Is this balance guaranteed? No, never, just a "hey we tried our best, and unfortunately the patient will just have to live with the results." If the result is death, "we are so sorry"; and if it is disability, "hey you may be in luck as at least some pharmaceutical companies may pay for your end stages of life healthcare needs." A nice stipend for covering clinical trial risks. But again, most vaccine liabilities are either wrapped into the cost of development, or if it gets approval from the FDA as a mass marketed drug, the VICP will begin to pick up the costs of litigation and settlements for such vaccine injuries. It is a sweet deal once you get the FDA approval to mass market a vaccine.

But does the government suggest they support vaccine approvals for mass production and distribution in all novel therapeutic and protective vaccines being researched? No, the government does not guarantee vaccine protections or liability; but openly suggests a safety net exists once a drug reaches the mass marketed status, and they will administer the safety net to ensure the vaccine is protected under the VICP program. Again, this is a discretionary approval process and a discretionary, administrative, and regulatory program, which have poor oversight and few constraints allowing poorly understood vaccines into the market with marginal safety recorded profiles. Science is not the primary concern, as many of the programs are designed to push and promote the vaccine drug class.

And the antibiotic manufacturers, what happened to them, since 1986 when the vaccines suddenly found some traction? Antibiotic research and development programs have consistently declined in the past few decades. First losing ground against bacteria-resistance problems, as doctors randomly and rampantly overprescribed antibiotics such that bacteria evolved and developed resistance because of such widespread prescribing practices. This may sound eerily like the overprescribing practices relating to synthetic opioids, which would also grow into an epidemic where the government and doctors are also guilty of mismanagement and application of drug laws. The road to improved antibiotic development has not been as smooth as many would hope and a lot of manufacturing has moved to lower-cost countries, so we do not have the key ingredients or the manufacturing capacities in our country we once had to develop new and better antibiotics.

Bacterial infections have also evolved and become more sophisticated, calling for a need for more sophisticated science. But is the funding there or is the interest in investing in antibiotic drug class on the decline? The answer is no the funding is not there, but manufacturers and researchers are always searching, and the best science does not often come from government scientists but from individuals, often individuals with specific interests and concerns. Antibiotics have fallen, but the antibiotic drug class is far from dead, as pharmaceutical experts have many tricks learned in slowing and killing bacterial pathogens, as we are smarter than a bacterium aren't we? Maybe, maybe not, as this is not a race being done at warp speed, but a slow and constantly changing infectious speed, concerning evolving bacteria and opportunistic pathogens not yet discovered (there are many), or ones that may evolve into an untreatable infectious plague or pandemic. Where the antibiotic manufacturers are not making many new discoveries, the vaccine manufacturers are happy to jump in and offer ideas. And why? Because government funded research opportunities and aggressive protection from liability if you have not already noticed the legal burdens being applied to different drug classes in the drug marketplace.

Complex problems require complex actions by the government, right? Not always, especially as the government is firmly wrapped into the promotional and commercial interests of vaccine drug manufacturers while offering suggestively "simple" vaccine solutions to the public. Sometimes the individual's pursuit of facts and evidence are the best option for public health concerns, as government authorities and manufacturers play information and fact-hiding facts games which are political and financially-driven, including selling off key pharmaceutical ingredients, and moving manufacturing to low cost countries with huge tax incentives. The public does not demand new vaccine standards for vaccine safety or reporting information regarding what the vaccine facts are today, instead looking to standards of the past as acceptable standards for the present and future vaccine safety concerns.

The fact many new novel vaccine therapeutic options have demonstrated and reported new observed ADRs more clearly documented than the older protective vaccine drug actions does not seem to fully register as an area of concern for most citizens, some citizens arguing vaccines are vaccines and all vaccines are expected to do the same thing, help the body's immune system develop antibodies to fight off unwanted infections and other unwanted "not normal, foreign" stuff circulating in the body. This is a potentially fatal flaw in vaccine safety practices as currently applied by many parties as being acceptable, using the suggestive benefits of vaccines while ignoring newfound vaccine ADRs. Making it an acceptable practice by Vaccine Inc to falsely endorse and promote vaccines through laws and agencies legislated as part of the Vaccine Act.

Which brings us to another prudent question that at some point must be addressed for all infectious disease "class" drugs, and that is when would it be appropriate to also give antibiotics, antivirals, and biologicals pharmaceutical manufacturers a protective liability umbrella as well. These therapeutic infectious disease drug treatments surely warrant additional liability protection to seek better infectious disease treatment drugs with little concerns for being sued. The path to better healthcare is surely driven by use of more legal protections given to medical professionals and pharmaceutical manufacturers, rather than to citizens, exempting parties in the masked names of public health and safety.

Suggesting more broadly defined exclusions from liabilities for more drugs are silly and nonsensical arguments. However, if citizens do not object to such constitution-bending exclusions and false safety nets in the name of healthcare, perhaps it is appropriate such exclusions will someday become more widely accepted and universally adopted. Drug and healthcare policies are complex public health issues, but drugs are a vital part of the healthcare system where drug costs may be rising but represent only a fraction of the overall healthcare costs. Low-cost drugs with no liability are a suggestive answer to out-of-control healthcare costs. Implied lower manufacturing and distribution costs of vaccines are not a good reason to protect any drug class from legal liability as being an unquestioned benefit to the public's overall healthcare cost and healthcare drug strategy for all citizens.

The costs of drug research and addressing medical safety concerns for citizens are of course an enormous cost to society. Citizens often blindly accept risks with limited to no facts to base a decision on regarding safety or effectiveness, as history has shown that citizens and medical professionals often overlook facts and information learned through science in hopes of finding answers and solutions to an immediate concerns. I wrap up this history section, not as it is a complete history of vaccines, infectious diseases, public health disasters, and such; but as a note to the public, as most Americans do not understand how the drugs work and the laws that govern drugs in our society.

In 1986, the vaccine law and drug laws in our country were quietly altered. It could be argued many parties claim awareness of the changes, but all citizens are sadly not prepared to acknowledge their lack of understanding of both vaccine science and the

Vaccine Act. Vaccines are no longer administered to citizens under normal food and drug (FDA) laws but fall under a far more special legal classification. Why is this important? Because the vaccine laws were never fully understood by most citizens? The lawyers who wrote the law, slanted it to protect vaccine manufacturers. There are few lawyers among citizens that understand the law and its ramifications, and even fewer that want to go practice law before the VICP special masters and judges. Especially about an off-Table injury claim, and especially regarding medical complications they have no educational training and limited medical understanding of being related to vaccines.

Lawyers, ever the protectionists of their flawed profession, will aggressively proclaim their profession sufficiently supervises all laws and aggressively advocates for all clients but there are fewer than 130 attorneys across the country in practice in the VICP Petitioner bar and I can attest few are strong advocates for their vaccine-injured clients or can claim understanding of the science.

These lawyers being the sole legal professionals authorized to practice in the VICP vaccine court, pretending they understand the Court rules, statutes, and regulations, and "how the court works". Most are elderly (many should be retired) attorneys with years of experience and a limited knowledge of the government's VICP courtroom players, with an understanding of court rules being their sole claim to applying successful arguments in the program, as they know a few special masters and quirky rules, which only goes so far when it comes time to argue science. By a legal standard, VICP lawyers are all professionally substandard attorneys in the practice of law, and completely incompetent regarding understanding science and vaccine facts, but certainly can follow a Table Injury matrix for a claim, if the vaccine injury claims is on the injury matrix.

By medical standards, the lawyers and politicians who wrote the Vaccine Act and the lawyers that now act as judges to protect the vaccine laws, sometimes being the same lawyers overseeing vaccine program development and safety oversight, would never pass any medical and certainly could not pass a pharmacy licensure tests if required to by some federal mandate, let alone understand the numerous statutes of drug laws found in each state's drug laws which are similar but different from federal law. Legal professionals are not paid to argue science or medical practices. Lawyers are paid to argue flawed legal logic and are suggested as an advocate for their client. Which is not just my opinion of how Vaccine Inc works today but has become an accepted standard among many parties.

Almost all vaccine claims lawyers fail to be effective lawyers and advocates for their vaccine injured clients. Where attorneys often raising stupid points of law or try to play vaccine courtroom playhouse drama rather than arguing science, and where appropriate documented science clearly cannot be addressed in a biased and foolish court. The arguments made by many parties are nonsensical legal games which are sporting gamesmanship played by lawyers, and not a scientific argument by any measures for addressing a vaccine-injury claim. Injured parties must accept suggested "fair" settlement, or get nothing, as the government has granted a special master judicial powers with the promises of fairness and justice, and the only party at risk of getting nothing is the injured party.

I think I have heard stories like this in evil fairytales, but the reality of the government's vaccine injury program is even more bizarre, as the parties being harmed are often children. Maybe scientists should create a vaccine to cure sick government authorities that come up with stupid ideas like creating laws that protect vaccine companies and paying friends and other legal professionals for administering the law, which often leads to far worse results for individuals and the public. I would pay to develop that vaccine. In fact, I have some ideas for developing the vaccine. Maybe the government will fund it? Since it would be a great vaccine and an incredible service to the public health, but maybe they would not like the adverse drug reactions which I am sure they would quickly add to the Vaccine Injury Table. The Vaccines Act makes us live in a bizarre drug world with disturbing medical consequences.

Many medical professionals have shifted their opinions of vaccines over the last 40 years, where many are now taught to be proponents arguing the promotional message for vaccine needs where public sentiment often lacks interest, where medical professionals with little interest in understanding core safety concerns, instead promote the government's recommended directives. Medical professionals do not ask about adverse side effects and risks, they simply refer to a CDC guideline and promotional literature supporting vaccines.

Medical professionals have also fallen victim to well-funded government public health department agendas, with a lot of government funding for promotional messages and training in an otherwise uninteresting public health profession. If you are a medical professional in need of a little extra income and would like to be viewed as a high-ranking public official, the field of public health may be for you. The public will offer their respect but few in the medical professions give much thought to such public health positions.

And the profession many citizens point to as being "the vaccinators", pharmacists, have shifted dramatically from being medical professional working as independent practitioners to being workers practicing inside a corporate shell, often bowing to the corporate pressures to mandate vaccines be administered as a business plan to generate more patient foot traffic to stores often with inflated priced goods. Insurance companies help with promotion as well, as the overall costs to insurance companies are reduced, and citizens are protected from some infectious diseases and the government picks up the liability cost expenses. It is a win-win-win-win… proposition for many parties. Why fight the system when the system pays the bills? A good question but at some point individually, or when someone you love is harmed, you will know my position, and it is the same position many citizens take for other causes and inequalities. I do not scream for justice, for justice has clearly failed and is not found for many individuals. I simply demand facts be addressed, so all citizens can learn, and maybe at some point justice will be granted in some fashion to those parties that have suffered or will suffer from vaccine injuries in the past, present and future.

Science is a vital element in understanding all drugs. If we do not follow the science in understanding actions of all drugs, we will never be fully safe, or make key discoveries that save and improve lives. We instead follow guidance from government sources of what they believe is best for the uninformed citizens, and certainly best for their selected interests decided by chosen authorities that may or may not know the science, or simply create a narrative and laws they believe is best for citizens. And what happens now if something goes amiss? The answer is nothing happens, as the government covering all the costs for errors and flawed laws, as all citizens must know by now, nothing ever happens to fix the existing state of affairs.

History is a critical piece of this discussion, as we will repeatedly be faced with important decisions of-the-moment in the face of infectious disease outbreaks, and even other everyday infections. Many people die from non-COVID/Influenza/Pneumonia infections, by either virus, or more commonly by bacteria, fungus, or worms? Cases known to be in the millions. Do we have therapeutic protocols to address all of these immediate concerns? The answer is no, not in all cases, as our government has failed to be prepared through gathering resources, logistical training, preparing protocols, and strategic preparations. Do we need to address all concerns with shutdowns and quarantines? Seems a little nonsensical, but many citizens have already learned to live a different lifestyle where the impact from stupid government actions are greatly lessened. We are on a never-ending journey which will not end with the current outbreak, and the answers to COVID and other infectious diseases will not be fully understood anytime soon. It is simply obligatory we learn our lessons, not just in science and medicine, but in laws and government practices. History offers lessons that are not just vital but mandatory, to learn how not to make the same mistakes repeatedly again-and-again. These laws affect all citizens' lives and the laws being practiced affect science. If the laws are not understood or are randomly enforced or discriminatory against any individual, the laws should be thrown out and granted to the citizens as lawful rights to demand information and the right to make informed consent decisions as prescribed by law and as understood through science.

CHAPTER 4

Just The Facts

Many readers will ask where I get my facts from for this book, and why should any citizen believe me, as opposed to believing our government. Surely the government has earned our trust. Yeah, right. The answer is rather simple. My facts and statements come from scientific research and my practice as a medical professional for decades. I have been around medical professionals, pharmaceutical professionals, finance, insurance, and medicine in general for decades. I know medical and drug law better than most lawyers, as very few know the fine details of drug laws in particular, and I can find the laws governing our drugs noted as being vague and discretionary or not worth arguing because they only exist to give judges and regulatory agencies discretion rather than address the real problems our healthcare system suffers from today. I can give lawyers and judges science and they will stand there with a dumb-look on their face, because it is science and commonsense, not law.

At some point, most scientists understand they will not get anywhere with nonsensical points of legal arguing in our lifetime. Maybe someone with a loader voice and more aggressive personality would be a better advocate for citizens, but I have given up on finding such a medical professional willing to step-up to the plate with facts and evidence. Perhaps, it is my duty to give the citizens the facts and evidence they need to understand what I believe is their legal right, but it is not a citizen's right if the citizen does not stand up for their rights. Science is vital and not based on my opinions or beliefs, as I am happy to share my facts and evidence, but I will not exhaust readers with science they do not care to learn or understand, or legal arguments which are boring. This book is based on facts and my experience, which you may find worthwhile, in judging for yourself, as to what is important and relevant concerns all citizens should have today, and certainly should consider going forward into the future in judging vaccines and healthcare options for infectious disease treatments.

Without science and discoveries, we must adapt our lives to fit "of-the-moment" emergencies and crises which can either turn out poorly or will naturally work themselves out. A natural progression with outcomes that happen which we have limited control over. I know most citizens learned this concept in school, but sciences are founded on observed facts and natural laws, not laws of opinions and beliefs. What group argues science? The government will argue they have the most science, which is piled deep and their selling it cheap if you have the time to review and read it. I will argue, I stand by science as discovered in textbooks, case reports, FDA pharmacovigilant reports, global studies, and independent and professional research by scientists for scientists. The vaccine facts are clear, and if you read facts and evidence presented by our government you will often find nonsense and generalized error-filled statements. I gave our government's vaccine experts and authorities science, and the VICP and government gave me nothing but stupidity and nonsense as its answers. You can suggest, I and other scientists are stupid or biased too, but I will open my vast volumes of facts, whereas the government stands empty handed, supported by a legion of authorities and medical professionals that only have an interest in promoting vaccines. I say the government should show its evidence to all citizens, I know they have a lot; and give heartfelt opinions on why they believe what they believe, as I will certainly be showing my facts and evidence and giving my opinions of where the government is wrong on facts, including some vaccine facts and evidence the government does not wish to show the public.

And evidence I present to citizens is not exclusive to my opinions, as our government has so nicely wrapped their strategy of justice around a few special masters randomly deciding facts and science to fit their legal point-of-view regarding vaccine-related injuries. You can find the special masters' and other judges' opinions and other agencies' opinions online and through government requests for documents if you have the time and interest. I find it more useful for citizens to share facts, facts citizens may not be aware of by any methods of research, but facts available in the public domain which are sometimes a little hard to bring together if you do not know the tools and request procedures. And facts you can only get from the source if the source cares to share.

Facts the government does not care to share, and many stupid parties, like attorneys, think they have access to, if they cared to see them, but they do not have access and therefore cannot share. Not that I have found many attorneys that would share if there were not some financial incentives involved. I like most citizens refuse to pay worthless legal professionals for pointless work when there are no repercussions for their inconsequential input of opinion. Our government does not grant open public access to any vaccine program files and vaccine injury claims, and the only party that has full access is the party that started a claim and followed through on it all the way to its end. I am one such individual, and I have records to fill a small warehouse. The government will offer facts and evidence in public judicial opinion statements, not in court records or in testimony. For that you need the source, and the source is documented in personal notes, legal records, transcripts, and filings to courts and agencies. In short, I offer facts. Our government offers opinions and flawed beliefs.

The Vaccine Injury Compensation Program (the VICP) was conceived as a shortened and abbreviated type of compensation program that prefers to have claimants settle injury claims based upon brief fill-in-the-blank science. Where even the government's experts have trouble interpreting and discussing the vaccine injury science or filling-in-the-blank. Does it help to have an expert who can explain the science, or a claimant that also understands the science? No, as the special master clearly has no clue following an expert's testimony what the science was, and a claimant who is not a physician cannot be permitted to give any clues of facts relating to the science. Most citizens would say, facts are facts, and evidence is evidence. No one can change that, except a bunch of Department of Justice lawyers, government experts, and special masters who like to form their own narrative and pursue a predetermined outcome. Claimants should not humiliate our government as our government does not like to look stupid.

The party claiming a vaccine injury (also called the claimant or petitioner) has only limited options to be heard in a VICP courtroom or any federal Court for that matter. I suggest other public forums not tied to the government would be a better choice to pursue a fair vaccine-injury claim. And I have learned after submitting multiple complaints and citizen petitions, and still waiting on several agencies to respond, where agencies often claim to be too busy to answer the petitions in a required timeframe which they set and cannot address my science or complaints I have outlined as important to science and citizens. So, rather than waiting on the government to address my concerns in a public forum, I am addressing my concerns in this book, and in an online website, under the Constitutional amendment allowing for freedom of speech. If my arguments are incorrect, and I say this to any party, simply show me the errors. As I would have settled my son's claims in the VICP in 2012, when the special master first offered to settle my claim for my son. The scientific evidence was not wrong in 2012 and was seriously twisted to fit a legal narrative in 2018. The facts were laid-out and understood and remain relevant today. The facts simply should be heard by the public and the public can do with them as they chose to do individually as citizens and parents. I suggest citizens act, as I can only inform citizens of facts and evidence. Citizens will need to take their own initiative and can adopt my plan of action which I believe is, a fair and just plan of action.

I stand in the same position now as many citizens who have gone to the VICP seeking settlement of a vaccine injury claim, and I have come out thinking does it really take that long to artfully craft a take-it-ot-leave-it settlement. Six years to a hearing, to hear bad experts explain false science, to twist medical records to fit their narrative, as the misinterpreted records did not even fit the claim. A stupid and twisted legal process, and a clear waste of time and money. I say these statements with no apologies, as any reasonable person could have explained the science in a simple sit-down meeting, which allegedly happened on several occasions between lawyers. The VICP program is a flawed suggested resolution game with multiple parties that do whatever they like, or as my stupid attorney, Mr. John F. McHugh, would always say, "it is what it is" and no one can change that, unless of course you are a lawyer and fail to do your job and give the other party discretionary room to make false decisions and flawed narratives, because you as the attorney failed to make the arguments by constantly stating "oh, it's okay the special master knows that fact" and "she understands the facts".

The claimant and the claimant's experts (me and my experts) were told we do not need to explain the facts or science further, as the special master already stated she understood the facts. It is clear she did not understand the facts or the science, and the facts and science really do not matter anyway. And the offers to settle are not real. The special master's decisions are completely discretionary. No real science or medical facts necessary, the biased final judicial opinion was decided before the trial even began. Vaccines win and citizens will lose, with or without scientific evidence.

It must be stated as it is perfectly clear many citizens have filed vaccine injury claims over the last few decades which were valid but wrongly determined by a special master as having insufficient evidence of a vaccine-related injury linked to timing or causational mechanisms. As a claimant you must satisfy the special master that both are relevant, and if they do not understand one, then they can also misunderstand the other. I can use science and pharmaceutical expertise to explain both, but the pharmaceutical science relating to drug actions are too much for many special masters. Our special master needed tea-party like discussions of science, with government experts that may as well have been drunk, as the experts and discussions reached seriously low levels of scientific discussion. I hope to allow citizens to see what the Supreme Court Justices clearly missed as a discretionary action in evaluating arguments of the lower VICP court, and to give citizens a fair view of what our government believes vaccine justice should be. I found vaccine justice to be stupid, nonsensical, and false with regards to science understood to be related to vaccines. Some would say, "accept defeat and move on", but I have already accepted defeat and the fact most parties in our legal system are scientific morons. I will move on but I move on with a purpose, and that purpose is to serve God, to serve my son, and to serve those who have been harmed by drugs of all types and cannot get their message heard as granted constitutional rights for justice and care by our fellow citizens. I will never be the voice of all citizens, but I can be the voice of citizens who are silenced and not given proper forums to discuss science and facts, and those that care to understand vaccine facts and our vaccine laws.

Many of my citizen actions are currently in process and future actions and statements will come in many formats, but my actions will be directed at giving citizens fair access to a fair forum to address vaccine injuries and a flawed vaccine law. One where citizens can display their VICP files for public viewing, at their discretion and not the government's discretion, which is currently noted as all VICP records are held as confidential, and the government suggests the VICP is a "secret court". So secret most citizens have no idea how it works, but citizens really should learn and understand the actions of our government's authorities, because as they say, it is the law and we are expected to understand the law. But how can citizens understand the law, when 99.99% citizens do not even understand the law exists or how it works? Highly educated doctors and pharmacists barely understand the law, and it is their job to understand our nation's drug and medical laws. I have had discussions with many other injured parties and not only are they disgruntled but also find facts and evidence of how the VICP court operates as nonsensical and harmful. I have read their vaccine injury claims, and many have been poorly addressed from a scientific standpoint. As any citizen that has gone to court knows, there is the law, and then there are the rules and court discretions permitted among lawyers and judges, where the interpretation of the law is mostly open to discretionary acts, and parties argue stupid opinions and beliefs in some suggestive antagonistic fashion, when the Vaccine Law clearly states it is legislated to favor the claimant regarding an injury "more likely than not to have been caused by the vaccine".

In the end, facts and science are always expected to win in any argument involving sciences, but vaccine injury arguments are not based on science but are based on discretionary understanding by multiple attorneys, including the one who is being paid to be the advocate for their client but somehow forgets to do their job. Again, no problem for the government, as the attorneys on all sides will still be paid in full for their legal time, services, travel, and extras. That is not discretionary, that is the law and lawyers will certainly fight for their money which the Vaccine Act states is due and must be paid, which also explains why cases are dragged out for many years, as more billable time equals more money and less effort by all attorneys involved.

I will provide my facts, opinions and perspective for those that care to hear the facts from my medical perspective and a few other experts, in an online forum, which I hope other parties will share their experiences related to vaccines as well. As they say more facts equals better results for everyone. I cannot change the science that dictates how a drug works or what actions a drug takes inside the human body, even as all government parties know vaccines certainly cause both known as well as less well-understood adverse vaccine injuries. The government however does not provide an open forum for public discussion of vaccine injuries which ultimately falls to the public to demand. The concerns for vaccine injuries may well sway many citizens now, as government actions related to vaccines will surely peak soon as the government attempts to convince citizens to overlook the vaccine drug class safety record which has been largely based on limited vaccine science. I know many medical professionals would completely agree with addressing any such vaccine injury concerns in an open forum and under a fair legal process, where all facts and concerns are laid-out to discuss and a fair jury decides the proper outcome.

Vaccines are a challenging drug subject, as vaccines safety concerns have never been at the forefront of discussions about vaccine injury mechanisms of causation. Vaccines injuries have been poorly reported as drug injuries which has been true since the days of variolation. Some vaccines are mature profiled drugs, with some well-understood complications. And some vaccines, like influenza, have had problems for over a century going back to when the flu vaccines were first developed. Yet still influenza vaccines continue to have poorly documented injury mechanisms of causation relating to why certain vaccines cause certain biological responses. To understand a vaccine adverse response sometimes it is necessary to go to a different set of drugs in a different drug class to address the adverse response to determine what is the causing mechanism, as other drugs have been better researched and have more complete drug safety profiles, where the science would leave the average or even above average judge out in the dark unless someone explains the science.

So, drug experts, if permitted and often they are NOT permitted, can explain vaccine science to a special master, but the science presented is often too complicated for the Court as it relates to a vaccine injury. To reconcile the gaps in understanding the science, the special master is given discretion through the Vaccine Act to form their own understanding of the science, which is usually remarkably misunderstood science by a judge. I still to this day, find the scientific standards of our Courts remarkably poor. I would have thought a higher level of discussion would be mandatory, as the Vaccine Act promised to be fair and address vaccine injuries from the claimant's point-of-view, since the claimant has to present facts and evidence to support their claim, which is certainly not true. And all citizens should know that science is not a legal concern in the VICP, as the government's medical experts are pushing the vaccines are "safe and effective drugs" narrative. Sympathy and empathy are not proper substitutes for medical facts and science. A deep understanding of medical facts does not happen, and citizens should know that before they accept their vaccination shots.

As I have stated, I have reached out and challenged many agencies (the FDA, DOJ, CDC, ACIP to name a few), at all levels from top to bottom, and I can give a fair and unbiased opinion that each and every vaccine-related agency generally has responded very lackadaisically, in fact I am not sure they really believe they serve the interests of citizens and certainly cannot carry on a discussion of vaccine science facts, often from a doctor-to-doctor point-of-view. Many times, appointed experts have started a circular discussion of stupid unsupported opinions, and when asked where I get my opinion from, I reference specific studies and case reports, or textbooks or professional references. Sometimes I am shocked to find they do not know what some of the science is, as it is their designated area of expertise. But often they have made a predetermined conclusion before the discussion even begins, which I have found to be a predetermined practice about vaccine discussions. Vaccine injuries are a broadly misunderstood and neglected science and one which leans to polar conclusions even when presented facts to support an adverse drug concern.

Numerous government authorities have stated they will get back with me on my questions and concerns, or they will have other experts in a workgroup review and get back with me, but such promises and statements of concern have failed every time. Not that I am not persistent and annoying, but well-paid and well-positioned government authorities and paid consultants have failed to come back even once with an argument regarding vaccine injury mechanisms of causation or questioning the validity of studies or case reports. And I know they are listening, as they know my name by now, some of us even having informal greetings and acknowledgements. Most citizens can detect a brushoff, but a scientific brushoff is that the right way to address questions of science? Yes, that is what happens when a well-informed scientist gets snubbed on a regular basis by many government authorities. My science apparently got lost in their staff's science stacks, or just filed with the rest of the complaints. Yet, at least I spoke with some extremely "high ranking" authorities and experts who seemed concerned but did not care to share their views or expertise to, you know, clear up the scientific concerns being discussed. Many agreed with my concerns and promised to get back with me but have never returned my requests for regulatory action. Maybe my scientific standards are too high for government authorities to address, as even drug laws state they must be addressed; or if they wanted to they could simply slide under the legal standards set in drug laws since they are the designated authoritative experts or at least someone given the title and power to make discretionary if not absolute decisions regarding drug and vaccine safety.

Maybe it is easier to hide and hope citizens will go away. Or maybe it is time for citizens to stand up and demand answers and facts related to vaccines, as many questions have developed since 1986, and even before then when pharmaceutical drug laws became more stringent and detailed, presumably to give authorities more discretionary authority to dictate what the government believes are safe choices for citizens, and the legislated promise to give all citizens a fair and just system to address their concerns.

I know, a little honey makes everything taste better, but in time honey turns to sugar, and not particularly good tasting sugar unless you melt the sugar again. But my point is, with time everything turns sour or off-tasting, and false claims the government sets out as true are truly sour as time has passed and a law's legislated intent has fallen flat on its vaccine face. I simply asked for transparency, and a party that will address the facts and science in a fair and understood forum, which our government has zero interest in providing such transparency regarding vaccines. But I can provide a forum where citizens can review my facts and see where the VICP program is false and flawed in practice and opinions, and where citizens can be directed to case records and show where experts on perhaps both sides are foolish or irresponsible as doctors in a courtroom setting or are often uncomfortable experts and/or unprepared fools; and where pharmacists and drug experts from academia or private industry have been BARRED from discussing science in the vaccine discussion forums, even as pharmacists are experts in drugs generally above the government's physician-restricted medical expertise regarding drug actions which are often not fully understood by doctors; and whereas doctors are given wide discretion to talk in speculative and grossly biased science which is both infuriating and absurd. Citizens should demand to hear vaccine-noted truths and facts of science. It would help citizens to understand the law and vaccine injuries, as many citizens simply do not understand the drugs, or the drug and medical laws.

I suggest, at some point in the near future, citizens will be shocked or unfortunately injured by a vaccine which can be explained as being a vaccine-related injury, and most likely could have been prevented if not for the prejudiced stance of our government. Actual vaccine-related injuries have been linked to many viral-based vaccines. I can list the vaccines here, but the most reported vaccine injuries are listed as being related to vaccines used for protection against viral infectious diseases. Influenza vaccines standout as a common troublemaker in VAERS reports and VICP claims, creating a lot of reported problems but are exceedingly poorly managed injury cases in the hands of biased authorities.

Perhaps the government is spreading out vaccine injuries before they are accepted into the Vaccine Injury Table, as GBS was recently added to the Vaccine Table Injury, as was SIRVA (an acronym for, Shoulder Injury Related to Vaccine Administration and other injection site adverse complications). GBS only took 50 years to be accepted as having an acceptable mechanism of causation to warrant listing on the HHS-approved Vaccine Injury Table of acceptable vaccine injuries, and if you have an old GBS claim which was not previously addressed from the days following the 1976 Swine flu influenza vaccine fiasco, you now have a short period of time to jump in line to file an updated claim. Many citizens likely do not understand GBS-related complications are now an accepted flu vaccine-related injury and their doctors may have been even less informed in understanding the accepted causal relationship. If you have GBS, you may want to check with a VICP petitioner attorney or file the injury claim yourself, but do not wait or you will miss the final cutoff to file a claim. And the VICP is not like some government programs requiring special forms to be filed to specific authorities or you get nothing, which is a more common government loophole found in many other legal claims' programs.

The VICP petitioner must simply file a petition for a claim for injury as being caused by the specified vaccine. VICP bar member attorneys will often gladly file these claims, as it is money in their pockets, and almost a prearranged settlement as it is on the VICP Vaccine Injury Table. The settlement amount for resolution of a vaccine injury causing GBS can be significant. Do not miss your opportunity to file a claim if you or someone you know has GBS more likely than not linked to an influenza vaccination. For SIRVA, the settlement amount is generally much lower, but also has a time limit for past claims. Any citizen that gets injured and has a permanent or unresolved vaccine injection site injury, which can be related to the vaccine itself or the vaccine being improperly administered are eligible for claims to the VICP. Attorneys should love these vaccine settlements as they are like a class action settlement, with little to no effort on their part. Paste facts, file to the court, and get paid. Easy money lawyers, so get in line.

Doctors will also like these accepted injury claims, as it requires minimal effort on their part as well. If you have GBS from an influenza vaccine or SIRVA from any vaccine, start the claim processes as soon as possible. Otherwise, you may forever miss out on an opportunity to file such claims for your injury. The government does not widely advertise these claims opportunities, and your doctor may or may not be helpful or understand the legal rules and deadlines. And for future reference, all citizens should keep these noted injuries (GBS and SIRVA) in mind, as they relate to vaccines, but not all parties are interested in addressing these concerns in a public forum.

Sometimes a citizen will be left out there all alone to address a vaccine injury, but unless you want to accept the injury as just an unfortunate event, take it upon yourself to file a claim ASAP. As your doctor may not want to have their name posted on a government website where others are left to assume they are antivax or oppose vaccines but are really only trying to help a patient resolve a Table related injury. It is an odd process for all parties, but again it was part of a doctor's accepted Oath to serve and protect all patients agreed to when entering the medical profession. Ask for help, and if one party cannot or will not help, ask other parties to help. You can start the claim without other parties if necessary, but a treating physician will be required at some point in the claim, and medical records will be required to confirm the injury as being related to the noted vaccine.

And, in the future, if you should find a need to file a claim relating to a COVID-19 vaccine, alone or in combination with other drugs or vaccines, the claim for injuries will get a little trickier, as the injury may be covered under an emergency coverage as decided under discretion by the Secretary of Health and Human Services; or a COVID-related injury may get pushed forward like GBS was pushed forward for several decades. Some claims, like COVID-19, will fit a similar adverse risk profile as influenza vaccines, but again the causational mechanism of the injury may be extended as not being fully understood for a long period of time and will be aggressively disputed by the Secretary's pack of DOJ attorneys if the claims volume and settlement demand claims are large or complex.

These are simply minor vaccine safety concerns you may say, but small concerns can grow into major problems (again, think of GBS) and are poorly addressed in a discretionary legal process. A major gaff or production error by any vaccine-associated party can lead to a large volume of claims, which would require further government actions to cover the large volume. As the VICP is funded through vaccine fees and several agency operations, which may be tested and would likely result in a long and drawn out process, if history is our guide to lessons learned in addressing other vaccine injuries. Sure, Congress can fund any gaps in coverage, but that is not a requirement in the Vaccine Act, and more of a discretionary action should there ever be a shortfall.

The government argues the VICP is an efficient program, as costs are wrapped around vaccine fees and multiple agency funding sources. Why argue with efficiency? Because efficiency should not be at the expense of any individual citizen and should not be for the benefit of commercial interests that provide limited safety and reporting of safety measures as required by drug laws. Government auditors, such as the Government Accountability Office have not found the vaccine programs out of compliance but often suggests the VICP program and court system are flawed in how they manage their actions with relationship to the intent of the Vaccine Act legislation, suggesting the vaccine program has many flaws. The program administrators, special masters, and review judges, can make claims of giving their best efforts to be fair and balanced, but what is fair and what is balanced in the hands of biased judges? And will this fair and balanced position hold the weight of a colossal vaccine injury claim avalanche, should a massive set of injuries from a novel vaccine ever be used as a mass market vaccine, which was approved for an emergency but causes serious injuries or vaccine related medical complications? I would suggest the VICP and our government agencies are not prepared to address such an avalanche of vaccine injury claims. Whether they are Table or off-Table vaccine injury claims. Or maybe everyone will just get a tax credit or government check as a "We are Sorry" settlement, which seems to be a standard method of settling large numbers of claims which are difficult to address in our government's bureaucratic system.

Do not worry, our government is good for it, whatever "it" may be. But I say do not count on any government action, and citizens must make their own decisions as to what is best for themselves and their children. There is a need to prepare citizens for what arguments may be ahead, and be prepared to argue whether a vaccine injury is related to a specific vaccine causational mechanisms of injury, as it will be suggested a citizen likely had other medical conditions or triggers which may have caused the injury, and would require a mandatory six months or more, just to see if the complications could be corrected by the doctors, before the vaccine injury claim even becomes relevant. And many treating physicians will have no idea what the vaccine injury may be and may not fully understand it was related in some way to the vaccine. Remember these are likely the same doctors that recommended you take the vaccine in the first place. Some will wrongly think they are in some fashion liable, as it is with other prescribed drugs and procedures, and will dismiss the injury claim as they do with normal medical practice liability lawsuits, probably under the standard advice of their attorney, who also have no understanding of the VICP claims process. All citizens must understand, medical and pharmaceutical liability lawsuits are complicated and requires a lot of science being understood by legal professionals just looking to make a buck. The VICP program is not a normal liability claims process and will be confused and intentionally messed up as few citizens care to learn about the vaccine law and the massive government programs improperly developed to addressed citizen concerns enacted as the Vaccine Act.

So, citizens should just call a vaccine attorney if they are injured by a vaccine, right? Sure, but there are fewer than 100 "active" VICP bar member lawyers nationwide, and many are incompetent, or fail to address all claims of injuries related to a vaccine. Many cherry-pick the claims they feel they are best trained to address, Do not expect the first of these select group of legal clowns you contact to address your vaccine injury if it is not a Table Injury. And if there are numerous vaccine injuries being claimed at one time, a run on the VICP could be like a run on the bank when everyone wants to withdraw and protect their money in a financial crisis, where unfortunately most of the banks are closed or no longer operating their business at full speed, or are simply highly selective in which cases they believe are most likely to be resolved with the least effort. Keep in mind a simple vaccine injury case can be resolved in a few months. Payouts can start around $25,000 to the injured patient and $25,000 to the attorney for marginal effort. This can sound like a bonanza for some individuals, but this sum will get an injured party nowhere nearly close to an amount needed to take care of a serious medical complication or lifetime disability.

Pain and suffering damage settlements are capped at $250,000 (not adjusted for inflation in decades), which is not a bad amount, if you are an older person. If you are a child, such a low settlement would be a joke, to address a significant injury that can last a lifetime as a devastating disability. The special master will test your financial skills, and even suggest a petitioner or attorney is being greedy, or the injury is not that serious comparing the injury to some other unrelated injury they read about somewhere. As an injury designated as a full disability by medical professionals and federal agencies, which will impact a person for the rest of their life, can be dismissed as simply being a residue (no big deal) of an unrelated injury which certainly was due to something else and not the vaccine-related injury. A special master on their own initiative can subjectively and randomly decide the noted injury is not related to a vaccine.

Special masters will challenge the logic of medicine, but for what purpose? I went through all these cycles of nonsensical discussions, as the VICP court special master accepted the claim as proven as more likely or than not caused by the vaccine immediately after filing the injury claim, which then went into a test of knowledge and facts for many years, only to find out facts and science really do not matter. What matters is what the special master thinks as to whether a claimant is playing fair and is making a fair demand for settlement, not what outside experts and medical professionals say is fair and paid in the healthcare marketplace by all citizens. I did not put forward random demands, as I let experts, as designated in government guidelines, address the demand costs needed for settlement. Or better yet, if we want to look for "fairness", as designated in the Vaccine Act, we should look to what public officials in government, like congressional representative and what would they get as fair medical treatment for their injuries and medical care while in and after leaving Congress. The cost of care for these "elite" citizens is outrageously high and yet perfectly acceptable in their little world of government elitist entitlements. The Vaccine Act does not make such broad assumptions, but simply states that whatever costs it may take to return a vaccine-injured patient back to as normal of a life as possible is fair. What citizens should know is that a special master who is a lawyer with no medical training or financial expertise will be making the discretionary decision of fair settlement for a vaccine injured individual who is often disabled and unable to speak for themselves. And to add to the sick joke of suggested settlement, all party's flunk basic finance and adjusting for inflation. Where they cannot make basic inflationary adjustments to anything except their salaries which are generously adjusted upward each year, generously adjusted for all parties except of course the injured party.

In my son's vaccine injury claim, the special master was **Laura Millman**. She was a long-time special master who suggested almost immediately our claim be settled early in 2012, and again after three years when she pushed the case to Life Care Planners (a person licensed to estimate future health and life care costs), as I had requested, and pushed before an outside arbitrator as an independent third-party to determine a fair life care plan. The Department of Justice however did not have an interest in settling, as they had a directive to argue all off-Table injury claims aggressively and without much concern for the injured party. For the record, the independent arbitrator agreed with us in an arbitration hearing in 2016, but the DOJ again did not budge. Were we being greedy? You be the judge. Ms. Millman agreed to the causation in 2012, and suggested my attorney, Michael Baseluos, draft a demand (payment request) for settlement. Mr. Baseluos was eager to settle, and suggested we accept a low settlement offer to expediate settlement, which would work with his schedule as he needed the money for his honeymoon. The suggested demand offer started near the bare minimums, as if all parties would say sorry, claim empathy and move on, which is a great idea, except the person filing a claim is the parent, and trying to ensure the injured party, a child, is properly taken care of as permitted under the vaccine law. I suggested experts in medical rehabilitation should determine the damages, as that would be a normal insurance or legal demand process, and is the stated process understood as acceptable by federal courts (i.e. the government wrote the rules on this settlement process, not me).

I also learned other VICP facts as I moved through the Courts, and I learned the VICP process has an exceptional lack of transparency. The special masters and lawyers try to hide discussions and agreements. A standard legal "matters" practice held behind the scenes to establish a set of facts nobody cares to share or put in writing, including several parties it would have been helpful to know had a prior history and legal battles regarding vaccines before going forward. Ms. Millman a graduate of a NYC night law school in 1976 moved from law school into government services and began her career with the Department of Justice, where she continued to work as a DOJ lawyer for 12 years. In this period, the government was also scrambling to address the Swine flu influenza vaccine fiasco. Ms. Millman played a key role in protecting the manufacturers and acting as a government attorney in Swine flu vaccine-related GBS cases, and then helped build on her experiences to help create the legislation that became the Vaccine Act as part of the team addressing the vaccine-injury compensation fiasco from the government's viewpoint.

One of Ms. Millman's vaccine rivals in the vaccine injuries debate was my expert, Dr. Joseph Bellanti, who was one of the medical doctors treating and making assessments of the cause of GBS in Swine flu patients at Fort Dix in 1976. Although I did not know it until after the trial, Ms. Millman and Dr. Bellanti had a long history of being adversaries. I would have absolutely stuck with Dr. Bellanti as my expert, as he is without a doubt an expert in Immunology, and one of the few doctors I could find with a concern for vaccine injuries, and did not care that the government treated vaccines as if nothing was going on. He knew the immune system concerns, and he genuinely cared about vaccine-related injury concerns. In fact, he has played the role of advocating for many vaccine injuries for many years, including the GBS influenza vaccine injury finally added to the Vaccine Injury Table in 2018. I truly admire Dr. Bellanti, his truth and commitment to long-term efforts to assist claimants in explaining vaccine injuries. As an ally, one would be proud to have Dr. Bellanti on their side, as he provided balance and science to our vaccine-injury argument.

Unfortunately, he and Ms. Millman were long-term rivals, as she worked a long time to defeat his position on GBS and flu vaccine-related injuries. She worked over 12 years in the DOJ on GBS vaccine cases helping in representing and defending the government in nine important cases that the government took over relating to the Swine flu fiasco. In total, almost 4000 injured citizens filed cases claiming that the Swine flu vaccine shots caused them to develop the debilitating nerve disease. But citizens should feel safer as Ms. Millman during her early days with the DOJ and VICP liked to think of herself as a "self-proclaimed health and medical junkie" (everyone should feel much safer now, a medical and vaccine junkie lawyer was on my son's vaccine-injury case), often expressing she had sincere concerns for injured patients following the enactment of the Vaccine Act, and suggested to her superiors she would be a good candidate for the role of a special master, which just for the record solving medical "mysteries" as a hobby or as part of some suggested legal job is not quite the same thing as being a scientists where such life-changing decisions are critical to a job being performed every day. But, apparently she impressed enough of her superiors with her work that she was appointed as one of the first VICP special masters, which the Vaccine Act designated as the highest roles an authority could be assigned relating to making decisions on how and what actions were fair in addressing vaccine injuries in any given assigned case.

If you were a medical professional in this timeframe, you may remember the Vaccine Act being enacted in 1986, and hearing the government's promises to make good on vaccine injuries, and you may still think the same wholesome vaccine compensation program exists in this same honest suggested format, but that fantasy VICP court does not exist today. Ms. Millman can be given recognition as an important legal player in helping set up the Vaccine Law and the VICP program and she helped in getting the program rolling for over its first 25 years. Her legal influence certainly has help make the VICP program the flawed and dysfunctional citizen-aid program it is today.

Ms. Millman's early VICP influence began in 1991, as it took a few years to roll over vaccine-injury cases from one set of federal Court cases to an independent VICP Court program. She has said her early VICP cases were easier, and perhaps fairer as she tried to be fair and compassionate. However, in 1995, the HHS Secretary decided to add a layer of protection against injury claims by creating a Vaccine Injury Table, which would serve as a matrix Injury template for claims. An injury listed on the Table would be easier for special masters to address, as the cause and timing would be defined by the Table. If the claim was off-Table, a different set of rules would apply and the petitioner filing the claim would have to prove the vaccine both caused and had specific timing relative to the vaccine-related injury creating a far greater medical and legal argument for many vaccine-related injuries. And in 1997, the Secretary further refined the Vaccine Table injury making the cases even more difficult to argue. These legal actions significantly changed the VICP, with little input from Congress, citizens, or medical professionals.

In truth, the special masters, a few reviewing judges, and the DOJ had largely taken over management of the vaccine injury program, with input from a review board of consulting doctors to address medical concerns. Not doctors like Dr. Bellanti of course, but one of those doctors on the VICP board for many years was Dr. Arnold I. Levinson. Dr. Levinson would later join the government's team of vaccine experts and would recruit fellow experts that would be willing to act as experts on behalf of the government, as many were already on the government payroll through vaccine funding and research. Clearly there is a lot of concealed partiality in the VICP program, but a strong vaccine preference is advocated as prerequisite for the legal sport of one-upmanship and drama. The government's vaccine parties often acting like there is a strong need to be adversaries in vaccine injury claims, when the Vaccine Act stated there would be no such harm or aggressive tactics applied to any vaccine injured claimant. The VICP was to be fair and unbiased in addressing the vaccine-injury claims, but all parties quickly took a detour which became less favorable options for claimants.

One could say, over the next few decades, the chickens were all in the pen, with several key hens and roosters knowing each other well, and what roles they must play before the public and claimants. The public has been presented a suggested "caring" system with "fair and balanced" payouts, and the occasional complete failures in justice, which may get fixed at some point in the future when the science would catch-up and the injury would be added to the Table. The VICP program has pushed farther away from settlements for off-Table vaccine injuries, as off-Table claims have now become almost impossible to settle and any reduced settlement automatically requires injured parties agree not to blame the vaccines for causing the vaccine-related injury. A suggestive, "we know vaccines cause adverse injuries", but by accepting a reduced settlement all claims of any harm caused by the vaccine are released of all liability. There are no other avenues for making a constitutionally fair vaccine injury claim. The VICP has become the sole legal court to settle a vaccine-related injury claim. The DOJ has mostly succeeded in fulfilling its long-term goal of changing the Vaccine Act's legislated intent to provide fairness to all claimants, with its internal stated goal of squashing all off-Table claims regardless of validity. Who will complain about these changes in the VICP program apart from a few injured parties, and most of them are not citizens, they are children? What a great DOJ we now have for our citizens and our citizens-to-be.

Minor vaccine injuries that are on the Vaccine Table have often been paid quickly and fairly. More significant injury claims often takes years to reach a hearing, and are not settled but are often dismissed as not being "more likely than not" or " a feather over 50% as being related to a vaccine". This suggested reduced standard of proof has grown in size to being a higher burden of proof in recent years. Sorry, you can be 50.000001% or more correct up to a trial hearing, but be found to be completely incorrect in a special master's twisted mind as they can change their mind and decided their understanding of facts and science are suddenly different and the claim is not valid after a court hearing. The standards of proof of vaccine injury causation and timing are constantly being pushed higher for claimants today. I was prepared to argue with a degree of certainty at above the "most likely" standard, being more likely above a more than 90% level of being factually correct, which is far above the 50% legal requirement. In fact, as a matter of timing and causation I am certain nothing else could have been the trigger for my son's relapse except for the influenza flu vaccine.

Special masters have wide-discretion to misinterpret medical facts and to misunderstand vaccine science which often leads to flawed opinions in judicial decisions. There is no required understanding of medical literature, or discussion with other federal agency experts to clarify vaccine argued science. In fact, the special master can add their own spin on science and declare newfangled interpretations of science in total disagreement with the VICP's sister agency the FDA. The VICP gives the special master an extraordinary platform to address vaccine injuries and harm to citizens using their own "branded" form of science, as they see fit in applying the science which does not need to be current or understood among scientists. FDA, vaccine manufacturer, and global vaccine regulatory agency science need not be given for evaluation of understood science. The special master controls what is and was is not allowed as science once the case goes to trial, which is an extraordinary breach of legal rights for any citizen filing a vaccine injury claim.

The level of bias, and Vaccine Inc party handholding, which goes on in the VICP and other programs relating to vaccines should be noted as being very disturbing. As noted, Dr. Levinson worked within the VICP, and also worked with Henry Schein, the largest vaccine distributor to doctors' offices, and also with other businesses that market and promote vaccines. Dr. Levinson's fellow vaccine expert colleague Dr. Kaplan was a fellow academic doctor at the University of Pennsylvania's Children's Hospital (also known as CHOP), where Dr. Kaplan also had many ties to vaccine manufacturers, including a close tie to Merck, a major vaccine manufacturer. I could go on with the vaccine-related affiliations, but the vaccine-industry linked ties between all parties are tightly-bound financially and I do not believe there is an unbiased party in the government's VICP vaccine professional lot.

Ms. Millman was clearly biased and had a long-running antagonistic relationship with Dr. Bellanti, as each had strongly opposing points-of-view about vaccine safety concerns. My son's vaccine trial was absurd, and I would welcome any outside viewpoints which would care to address the many absurdities our government has deemed as appropriate in a court of law. Conflicts of interests and vaccine bias are one thing and should have been hammered out prior to any trial where conflicts of interests should be transparent to all parties, which are instead hidden as being unimportant to the least informed party, the injured party, and often the parents representing them. In the real world, the number of vaccine-injury interested parties is too small and are by nature biased in their opinions about vaccine injuries. A truly independent jury would have been fairer arbiters of what was valid and what was fair, but such jury-based fairness is not allowed under the Vaccine Act.

If we go back to 2012, the year I filed a vaccine injury claim for my son, Mr. Michael Baseluos suggested we not be pushy, as Ms. Millman was "on our side". In fact many VICP attorneys over several years would suggest Ms. Millman was a "fair" (yet no lawyer would define fair) special master, or at least less heartless than other special masters, some special masters being noted by vaccine attorneys as being extremely harsh and ruthless on vaccine claims, which I found a little odd. I reviewed numerous other VICP vaccine injury cases that had special masters that had trouble determining causational mechanisms, but I considered my son's case as being well supported by scientists and global nephrologists as influenza vaccines are a noted common trigger for nephrotic relapses, and such relapses could lead to further serious complications in treatment protocols.

Other VICP petitioner attorneys frequently noted Ms. Millman as being a little crazy and kooky at times, which I did not understand craziness as being better than the alternatives when one begins to talk about science as an argument. In 2012, Mr. Baseluos, our initial attorney, suggested he had a short timeline to address my son's claim, but despite his suggested need to rush a settlement I stood by our demand to have as many medical experts as necessary decide an appropriate settlement amount, and not just pulling out a number Mr. Baseluos felt would be a "good number". From a client perspective, it was like being in a car accident and the attorney telling you the other party agrees it was their fault, now how much cash do you want to settle? I had no idea, but it was not a dent removal case. I expected expert guidance, and all I received was a grade school level offer to make a trade. What is your child's life worth? More than $50,000, which is what a citizen may get in a vaccine injury case that causes death. My child was not dead, thank god, but his injury was profoundly serious. Mr. Baseluos was released from his attorney duties and freed to go on his honeymoon, with payments issued promptly by Ms. Millman to pay for his legal services. Likely paying for his wedding and honeymoon. Over $25,000 in paid legal fees for nominal legal services and a few meetings with Ms. Millman, but she liked him calling him a "good boy" on several occasions.

Mr. Baseluos did marginal work, which I later learned was a standard practice among many VICP bar attorneys as a substandard vaccine court legal representation practice. Again, there are 130 or so vaccine bar attorneys nationwide and I found none of them particularly impressive as lawyers, and even fewer knew what the nephrotic medical condition was or how it may relate to vaccine injuries. Attorneys that understand what nephrotic syndrome is as a medical condition falls into the 3 to 5 number range of VICP attorneys with basic knowledge of the injury, so a vaccine injured claimants cannot be picky regarding other attorney skill deficiencies, which I only state as some attorneys laughed (yes that is rude) and say we got what we paid for in selecting a substandard VICP attorney. This coming from a number of non-vaccine bar attorneys that fail to understand there are very few attorneys to choose from, without taking the quality of the attorney's education and professionalism into consideration.

Our next attorney was equally substandard, but recommended by a highly regarded law professor, Peter Meyers, of George Washington Law School in Washington D.C., a law school that operates a vaccine law clinic that tries to develop VICP attorneys who want to learn more about the vaccine program and its odd ways. Mr. Meyers no longer runs the legal clinic program as he decided working on the vaccine program was too complicated and flaws in the program would not be decided through the proper legal channels offered in our courts. He authored a long paper on the flaws of the VICP. I suggest readers look it up online or ask me and I will send a copy to you. Mr. Meyers later suggested appeals filed against a flawed decision and the likelihood the Supreme Court would hear the case were minimal based on those courts' prior decisions. In his professional opinion, the special master must be exceptionally arbitrary and capricious, meaning her opinions had to be exceptionally flawed and biased, which I could show her decision was full of errors and flawed and proceeded to file the claims myself, helping a fully disabled citizen make a legal claim using legal guides and textbooks that attorneys learn from in law school to learn and walk through the steps of filing for a review and a writ of certiorari in the Supreme Court.

I found out as I proceeded, much as I was told, that few judges or Justices cared to address flawed decisions from the VICP vaccine court, and most certainly not ones submitted by non-legal professional individuals. I found Ms. Millman's decision having over 100+ errors in science, giving preferential reference to multiple perjured expert statements by the government's experts, misunderstood causational mechanisms, misused medical records and child recorded logs, and many other flaws in her trial process seemed like a reasonable request to ask the Courts to rehear the evidence, as her interpretations were clearly wrong. Not in an unfortunate way, but as a very flawed and damaging way, as if she intentionally made flawed choices to harm my son's case to fulfill her pre-trial threat to accept her offer to settle for some "imaginary" settlement amount or else she would give him nothing, which is in fact extraordinarily biased and inappropriate as a starting point to a trial.

The only problem with her pre-trial threat was neither she or the DOJ attorneys had any defined settlement number, and our only number was the settlement offer her trusted nurse friend had given us which I had professionally addressed and calculated using proper financial adjustments as outlined in the Federal Justice Center guidelines for proper settlement guidelines and appropriate financial adjustments which are available to all citizens online, but as the DOJ did not address and refused to issue a valid offer, the "mandatory recommended" settlement to the case could not be resolved through any reasonable methods. Yet Ms. Millman could have suggestively forced a settlement if she wanted to, but even she did not know what the settlement number should be, as her preferred government-contracted nurse consultant did not give factual and defined numbers to settle. Many outside professionals suggested this scenario was highly unusual, but those that knew her stated with Ms. Millman anything was possible, and tactics used by the DOJ were strange but not completely out-of-the-norm. Apparently, petitioners (the injured party) must in some fashion reconcile and agree with the special master's point-of-view and be very agreeable in the courtroom or else suffer their wrath of pretrial threats which are often baseless demands in determining a real settlement.

The nonsense of addressing the earlier settlement and working with medical experts, hiring top experts in their field, and establishing a demand before an independent and qualified arbitrator was agreed with as a fair process by us, but was insufficient for Ms.

Millman. She had a different number in her head, and that number was more of a welfare number, except she did not understand, despite years of being a special master, the program cannot issue a settlement that uses funds from both the VICP and the Social Security and welfare programs. She had in her mind some blended settlement which simply could not be done and was restricted by other laws, so as the DOJ did not want to supply an actual settlement dollar figure, we simply had to go to trial. Why not, we had the science and the facts, why not prove the case in a real courtroom.

However, as I learned, after a flawed VICP hearing and decision, the only appeals process accepted are if the special master is in some manner overly arbitrary and capricious, which in the vaccine court is held at an exceedingly high standard of being offensive and biased in the decision on the claim. Facts like, science, getting evidence and facts wrong, and other generally offensive acts are all okay, if the special master was properly nice, which Ms. Millman would know since she helped write the VICP court's rules. I discovered and hopefully can share with all citizens that the VICP and special masters in the VICP, along with judges and Supreme Court Justices that have oversight of the vaccine program are, without a doubt, legal jokers regarding vaccines. I honestly cannot give a single recommendation to any of the lawyers that acts to represents VICP claimants, or DOJ attorneys that defend the vaccines and the HHS, to anyone looking for even an average attorney. I cannot say any one special master is exceptional in their opinions and understanding of vaccine science. I cannot say any appellate judge cares to understand the flaws in vaccine cases, in fact adding to the flaws in their opinions and in understanding the science. And the Supreme Court Justices simply dismiss any interest in hearing vaccine-related cases, as a 100+ year old Supreme Court decision serves as precedent for cases attempting to address and invalidity the Vaccine Act of 1986. I had been told by Supreme Court bar member attorneys, the Justices have no interest in vaccine cases, and have pointed to Justice comments pointing to the need for Congress to address the Vaccine Act as the only path to resolving any VICP court injustices, which sounds like a Supreme Court that no longer cares to properly address our constitution and individual rights, but prefers to allow laws and precedent based on political discretions, which I found unsettling but not entirely unexpected. The Supreme Court does not make the laws. The Justices interpret the validity of laws under their discretion, which clearly in cases involving vaccines they use their discretion to not address facts and evidence, as well as discriminatory acts against a disabled citizen.

I took my son's case to the Supreme Court because I was right on the facts and science, and my son had a valid vaccine-related injury as outlined in the Vaccine Act. The federal judicial parties just do not care to address these concerns, and all citizens should understand there is only limited interest in running a valid scientific-based VICP court as a method of resolving vaccine injuries. The court is flawed and harmful and cannot be trusted to make fair judgments as promised to address vaccine injuries. I would not have believed our courts handle vaccine injuries the way they do, if not for the fact I had the unfortunate opportunity to walk through the legal process myself, for my child. I do not recommend any exceptional steps be taken to improve outcomes other than taking the same steps I have taken may result in a similar unfavorable result, for yourself or your loved one. I would suggest vaccine injured citizens find other paths to settle a claim, in a different court if possible (which is not possible unless other drugs are involved), as my son's case was unique and had other liability issues relating to the treatment plan used following his highly complex vaccine-induced relapse complications, which not only did the courts screw up in the VICP case, but also screwed up his opportunity to seek a claim against the pharmaceutical company that contributed to harming him following the vaccine injury complications, which for the record are covered under the Vaccine Act but only if the special masters can understand the science, and they clearly did not care to understand drug science related to medical causational mechanisms that are understood in science today as the cause of many vaccine injury claims.

Addressing my son's other claim in a state court is complicated by the VICP program. In fact, the VICP makes the claim almost impossible, as it contributes to lawyers misunderstanding and reading of facts which they believe points to the vaccine-related injury, and believe a jury would blame the vaccine as the causative liability product. Vaccine-related medical cases are limited in scope, and few attorneys want to spend the time and effort to address a single individual's claim, as most prefer the class action shared-expense business model for making a living, rather than the justice needed for a single disabled individual. Disabled citizens are also dismissed or outright given no attention with regards to their unique professional legal needs for aid and advocacy. No attorney jumps forward to help a disabled individual who has a communicative disability which is specifically covered under ADA accommodations. Most lawyers make little to no effort to address the need for ADA accommodations, simply suggesting they cannot help or simply hanging up on the disabled party. What a shameful profession lawyers operate suggesting they serve all citizens needing help in seeking justice, but in fact their actions are far different from their claims to help those that cannot help themselves seek justice. I suggest most lawyers are disgraceful in their practices as professionals.

Which leads me back to my lawyers in the VICP, I accepted Mr. Meyers recommendation and hired Mr. John F. McHugh, who I was told was experienced and familiar with the VICP program as it sounded to Mr. Meyers that Mr. Baseluos was simply not experienced enough in the VICP and perhaps did not know "the players". In retrospect, many attorneys have suggested they are better attorneys than the VICP attorneys currently available to choose from in the VICP bar. Mr. McHugh suggested he had an extensive VICP program engagement experience and familiarity with the special master, which I assumed was professional. Later, after the trail, he informed me, he had a more personal relationship with special master Laura Millman, which I must state was rather an odd moment. Finding out your hired advocate had in fact had a personal relationship with the special master on my son's case. Yet another conflicting oddity in our government's little VICP vaccine world.

I accepted Mr. McHugh's early guidance as a client, but eventually discovered he had no idea what mechanisms caused the vaccine injury in my son's medical condition and even with tons of facts and evidence he still struggled with the facts and evidence when it was his time to advocate for his client in the courtroom. My family and my medical experts were astounded at how poorly he was prepared for the trial. In the courtroom Mr. McHugh is a featherweight who was more interested in playing it light on Ms. Millman rather than pushing for a hard discussion of science mandated for the case and for science in general, as our arguments were presented as being based on FDA statements and textbooks, in addition to case reports, peer-reviewed studies, and a nephrotic poster statement by experts in the field of nephrology stating plainly "Vaccines can trigger nephrotic relapses". The science on vaccines being a trigger of nephrotic relapses was and is credibly clear.

Mr. McHugh did not further explain his personal history until after the trial and during our heated discussions over post-trial briefs that he and Ms. Millman were in some fashion past close friends and in his eyes. Ms. Millman was a "delicate flower and getting ready to retire". Stating, he would never attack his "sweetheart", which would have been nice to know before the trial, because his sweetheart did not know her science. A lawyer is supposed to be an advocate for their client. Mr. McHugh is not an advocate for his client, in fact he probably should not even be practicing law, as his legal skills rapidly declined over the last few years prior to the trial, and would not be practicing law if it were up to me, but the NYC bar and grievance boards like to protect their own, so clients beware.

The state oversight agencies for lawyers are never on the side of an attorney's clients except in extreme cases, or as a manner of disciplining an attorney who is disrespectful to other attorneys. Legal professionals proclaim a required professional advocacy duty in representing their clients, while also playing footsie with the judges, which legal professional disciplinary boards consider perfectly okay. Attorneys do that all the time, its normal. The inappropriate things citizens learn about lawyers in our federal courts system are very odd and should not be accepted as being within the acceptable limits of professional practices.

As stated before, Ms. Millman was okay with granting a settlement in 2012, but I did not budge stating a need for medical and financial experts I believed were essential to determine our settlement demand, and after two expert reports in 2013 and 2014 Ms. Millman still stood on our side, and demanded the parties settle. Offering her preferred life care planner, Laura Fox, a longtime nurse friend and a contracted government supplier of life care plans to figure out a fair settlement. We hired Dr. Jane Mattson, a highly respected life care planner as recommended by experts at Deloitte Consulting, a top consulting firm. The two life care planning experts put together their settlement offers, both planners agreeing the same level of care was needed for future life and medical care. Mrs. Fox suggesting, she had consulted an out-of-town (but in-state) facility and believed it would provide the best future care for our son.

As part of the negotiations, in our arguments, we supplied three additional facility options as providing the best options for future care, as would be the standard steps and protocol in a normal insurance claim. Mrs. Fox flunked her required assignment on multiple points of proper settlement, including the simple task of contacting the facility she was suggesting as a fair cost solution. We contacted the same facility and received a quote substantially higher than her offered numbers, which we presented to an independent arbitrator. An outside independent arbitrator agreed with us, but the DOJ again refused to budge, under a higher DOJ directive to fight the claim at all cost. Who made this DOJ directive? It is uncertain and the DOJ's lead attorney Darryl Wishard would not say, as Mr. Wishard simply followed orders and directives to win at-all-costs, but the DOJ has a clear directive issued by some higher officials to fight all off-Table claims at-all-costs, as this directive is found on their website proudly proclaiming their stated objective and goal of seeking to eliminate all off-Table claims, and proudly suggesting they are close to reaching their goals.

Again, the DOJ finds off-Table claims to be a threat to the program and will do whatever it can to defeat such claims, but does this directive match up to the Vaccine Act's legislated intent. I would suggest it does not and does not match the intent in the way most citizens would read it, including the medical professionals openly promoting vaccines as being safe and effective, and in some fashion covered by the VICP program, but where an authority or authorities in our government or DOJ made such a directive and changed the shift in how the program would be run? Was it made in 1986, 1991, 1995, 1997 or 2016? Nobody seems to know, and the DOJ refuses to show such facts. In fact, the DOJ will not disclose any internal facts and discussions on vaccine claims cases, as these are internal DOJ affairs, not public records open for public discussion.

Citizens and lawyers can ask, but I find it a closed inquiry, as I do not have resources to fight that legal battle. So, a fair system and application of the Vaccine Law is no longer a valid path to resolving a vaccine-related injury. Our vaccine justice system works against citizens behind closed doors, and citizens really have limited paths to seek fairness or justice. We, in isolation, had two options, accept a settlement offered randomly which was the figment of a special master's thinking or fight the DOJ on facts and science. We chose to show the facts and evidence to prove our case, which even without including the science showed the government's expert were clearly lying and giving perjured testimony. I hoped to at least set some standard for future injured children suffering the same type of vaccine injury, but I did not understanding at the time there is rarely any precedent set by any special master.

Each special master it turns out can come to completely different conclusions based on the same type of evidence and arguments. Facts a special master sets as evidence from one case does not carry over to similar facts presented to a different special master in a different vaccine injury case, even as the cases are within a year of each other. The vaccine science is simply too complex for either special master and each special master was given wide discretion to misunderstand and accept false testimony by the government's experts. I can only restate, the VICP court program offers very odd interpretations of the Vaccine Law, and openly violates a need to address understood facts learned in science and explained in medical literature.

The peculiar part is Mr. McHugh clearly did not understand the science and causational mechanisms from 2014-2017 but continued and largely succeeded in working his personal relationship with Ms. Millman. Mr. McHugh's main problem being the DOJ would not budge, and Ms. Millman did not care to grant a request for more experts as would be normally be needed in a normal court trial. Ms. Millman felt she was the expert on vaccine matters (remember she is a self-proclaimed medical junkie) and her friends of the court, like Mrs. Fox would give her the guidance she needed, although Mrs. Fox was only a nurse and author of a government guide on life care planning (or LCP). For fun, ask your doctor how many LCP professionals they know, and most will say none. It is a field with many cross-disciplines of knowledge, which fits my area of knowledge perfectly. But apparently, we were not looking for a fair market-based settlement demand, we were supposed to be looking for a cheap low-cost settlement demand which would be more in line with welfare.

Ms. Millman, despite being in the VICP since its launch, did not understand a claimant cannot double-dip, or get a settlement and receive welfare payments at the same time as part of the settlement. A sticking point where it is clear special masters are not trained or experts in anything beyond their little world of legal discretions and opinions which are theirs alone, as again they do not have to follow any guidance from other special masters, or even other federal agency guidelines. The VICP court decisions are not precedent setting decisions, and the higher federal Courts do not care to give them any weight. The federal and Supreme Courts simply want to keep the VICP decisions in-house, and not assigning any failure to the VICP program and its flawed discretions. And who will show the Courts and our government that they have failed, if no one can see the facts and evidence? I will share the court submitted evidence and facts, and you can decide what should have been fair for a child with an injury caused by a vaccine and had major complications which did not resolve themselves leading to a serious long-term disability. A significant and accepted vaccine injury under the Vaccine Act. Any citizen can check it out. The Vaccine Act and VICP program rules and guidelines are online for any citizen to read.

Just do not expect everyone in Vaccine Inc to follow the laws and court rules exactly as vaguely presented in the law.

Today, Mr. McHugh still drifts around (or perhaps it is a senior citizen thing) attempting to find his next victim for filing a VICP claim to supplement his retirement funds, even as he should be kicked out of his profession. What client would want a lawyer who makes outright lies, misstates his ability, and files incorrect information in post-trial filings. I handled my son's case, providing the evidence and facts which were clear, and the Vaccine Act is not complex, but he clearly did not do his job as an attorney advocating for his client, my son, and gave Ms. Millman wide discretion to make clearly flawed decisions, which were distortions of facts and science.

How I ask did a law become so distorted and misused in such a short timeframe? If citizens consider our government today, all parties who represent the voice of our government do not care about facts or evidence but have preferred outcomes they seek as government employees and experts being paid by our government, and focus on the need to stick to a status quo statement of priorities which are vaccines are more important than the safety and harm that may be caused to any one individual.

So where does the Vaccine Act stand in relationship to other Laws in our country? I would say exceedingly high on the list of all laws as relating to its importance as a law. Most citizens believe our laws require fairness and justice for all citizens, including our children. The Vaccine Act is not fair or just, and stands above several laws, including the FDA and ADA laws for sure. And the Vaccine Act is above or on par with many vital constitutional rights, as being more important than an individual's right to make informed decisions. I can clearly state without a shadow of worry that I am correct in my filed petition for my son's vaccine injury claim, but our government has adopted a Vaccine Law which is both harmful to citizens and harmful to science.

I could devote volumes of books on all the foolishness that swirls around the vaccine court and the VICP, but it would also demand volumes of failures by many agencies wrapped into Vaccine Inc both in our government and industrywide. As a full disclosure, I am not a simple ordinary pharmacist, and I do not ask readers or anyone to understand the deep science facts but should understand the deep flaws of our government's actions and legal entanglements they have developed to protect vaccine manufacturers and the vaccine drug-class. The Vaccine Act is not a fair or balanced law, as it has changed considerably since it was enacted, and not with input from citizens on all sides. Citizens should be sickened by our government's harmful tactics and their irregular approach to science. You can decide for yourself what actions you chose to make to demand changes which may affect your life as it relates to drug choices and drug safety.

Ms. Millman stated her preference to settle my son's case when submitted to the VICP in 2012, and perhaps did not care to go against Dr. Bellanti in 2013. As he laid out most of the science and facts in his expert statement letter to the court. She did not question the facts or evidence, in fact she agreed with them. Which later led to the threat, not a request, to settle or else, prior to trial. If a threat is not bias, what is? Judges are often biased, but there must be methods to seek remedy and the federal Courts offer no remedies, but instead endorse discretion as their accepted legal practice. I say this was harmful not just for my son's case, but for many vaccine injuries cases I have read and reviewed. The VICP program is reckless, and unfortunately reckless against children and disabled citizens which is wrong, which I firmly state as my professional point-of-view.

As a witness to this fiasco, and knowing what I know about other vaccine fiascos, I believe all citizens must consider not only the professionalism of our government and courts, but also their intended actions which are harmful to citizens. I ask citizens to think before they vaccinate and be sure you want to deal with a legal reconciliation program that does not act like a court or legal program for injured individuals but acts as a group of little tyrants with twisted personal agendas and a need to promote vaccines as a required protective infectious treatment. Our society should not be playing such foolish games with our citizens, especially with our children.

Citizens going into the VICP program must understand the balance of justice is not on the side of science, or on the side of the injured party, but is tilted by special masters and a Vaccine Injury Table where science is randomly updated every few decades or so. Fairness in application of the law is not discussed but is replaced by ignorant suggestions of discretion to a single judge for a case, where the constitution clearly states a trial by jury is mandated. I would not recommend any citizen try to present facts or science in this cruel court, as the court is scientifically incompetent. Why even try to offer science when the legacy of our government is to protect vaccine manufacturers and the implied effectiveness of vaccines, and vaccine injuries are played with as tools to manipulate the citizens, and not just the foolish citizens who do not know better, but also the medical professionals who are foolish enough to believe a real process of government protection exists for patients who are harmed. Medical professionals have zero incentives in addressing the needs of their patients, as there is zero concern for liability by any party, which is wrong as a professional standard and is wrong as a law and legal process under our constitution.

Several attorneys and citizens I have spoken to have suggested the standard set for addressing a vaccine injury is currently set too high for any special master or judge to understand a complicated case, and for most petitioners (the vaccine-injured parties) to be required to explain. I simply say the standard is not too high as there was not even a fair standard to begin with, as a simple promise enacted as a law changed and was twisted to see how long and what changes would be accepted by citizens before citizens would finally step-up and say no more. Federal judges and special masters do not understand the science, and do not care to fully address vaccine injury concerns. Again, I must ask, is this what citizens and parents of children accept as their level of protection for the vaccine drug class? Vaccines have been documented as causing vaccine-related injuries for decades. The government, with the help of Ms. Millman and others, have simply acted to aid manufacturers in hiding these concerns from the public.

As I am not sure if this is a collective action or a concerted effort to promote vaccines as being safe, without fully addressing both safety and effectiveness. I find it exceptionally unusual, our government and media jump on a vaccine's declaration of being effective on its path to seeking approval, and make little effort to address adverse safety concerns, as if no adverse safety concerns even exist for vaccines. This is not 1795, or 1976, or 1986 for that matter. This is 2020, and science should and must come first. Our children and future generations are counting on us to make good choices for them medically and financially, as our government does not take proper actions on all accounts with relationship to vaccines.

As a medical professional, I am asked to promote vaccines with a flawed safety evaluation and must give an incomplete required consultation before each vaccination. We should freely vaccinate citizens we are told as the CDC recommends it is the best choice. Do citizens really trust the CDC? I personally and professionally do not trust the CDC. In fact, CDC statements have been vague and mysteriously off track for years, often reflecting a designated political promotional agenda, rather than a scientific understanding of vaccine concerns. I have been told the science is there and the safety concerns are "minor", but this is the position authorities and doctors try to use to promote vaccines today, not a need or requirement to address vaccine safety concerns.

Not all doctors ignore vaccine injury risks, but many willingly accept the task of vaccinating as a professional duty that they believe has in some fashion been mandated. Forsaking the Hippocratic Oath each medical professional took upon entering the calling to practice medicine. Briefly noted as stating, "*I swear to fulfill, to the best of my ability and judgment, this covenant: I will respect the hard-won scientific gains of those physicians in whose steps I walk, and gladly share such knowledge as is mine with those who are to follow.*"

This is not just the Oath followed by physicians, but the Oath followed by all medical professionals. Many doctors just no longer follow their sworn Oath as it was originally presented upon entering the profession with the promise to cause no unwarranted harm to any patient, if empowered with the knowledge to prevent such harm. And to use medicine to promote good health for all. Medical and pharmacy students take this Oath to "first, do no harm". Yet somehow this oath gets replaced with a required need to take steps that will cause no harm to themself or their practice and more specifically to take whatever steps are necessary to avoid getting sued.

Citizens must understand there are hidden harms in healthcare practices, which are not fully addressed in our current medical and legal system. Vaccines cause harm to patients, but there is no implied liability for such damage caused to the patient. Should we blindly recommend drugs that have no liability and provide all connected-parties absolute immunity? The answer for most medical professionals is simple, they must follow recommended government guidelines and avoid becoming involved in the discussions that swirl around vaccines and vaccine injuries. A sly but understood requirement to protect vaccines, or if vaccines were to ever lose their liability protection, medical professionals may also lose their protections from liability relating to vaccines.

I can confidently affirm lies and perjury are acceptable professional practices by medical professionals in the vaccine court, and the perjury by the government's expert witness who actively act as the government's voice. I will discuss these actions later, and more completely online in a website dedicated to vaccine facts and evidence, not just relating to my son's case, but I hope with facts many citizens who have gone through the VICP experience can also offer to share their encounters. I hope arguments can deal with both positive and negative aspects of the vaccine program and address its many flaws. Citizens should not be forced to accept an injury settlement they are pushed into accepting or feel they are powerless to fight against our government as they do not have the knowledge or the resources to fight our government's vaccine program and agencies. Fighting is not always the best choice, but sometimes even if you lose in a courtroom, you fight on. As there are simply too many wrongs falsely being suggested as being addressed in the vaccine programs, where a negative plus a negative does not equal a positive, as that logic only works in multiplication and division. Simply removing one negative aspect of vaccine programs and oversight is not going to balance the discussion of harmful actions by our government. The only real option is to remove all negative concerns and potential harm to all patients, as an oath I pledged as a medical professional I would always do for all patients. Understand and using drug facts and drug science as vital arguments which must be open to discussion among all citizens including scientists and medical professionals.

My facts will be posted online at www.VNTY.Health. Please request references to facts and ask relevant questions you may have about my statements and facts. I hope these facts, resources and discussion are helpful to other citizens to make informed vaccine decisions. I am a medical professional and I routinely share facts and knowledge with other medical professionals and the public. My peace is found in safeguarding my family and members of society. Perhaps a time will come where citizens put an end to discretionary justice, and demand real justice for all citizens that are not treated fairly under our legal system or are not given justice in a fair setting. There is no room for bias in our laws, and if a scientist is wrong, the scientist should openly admit such error, or at least acknowledge their errors in understanding the science. Whenever possible, I demand and ask for science, and suggest citizens should demand science as related to documented science, not statements of experts who proclaim they are the science experts, and they alone control the understood science message. An expert's message can often be false, must be challenged, and validated.

I will give facts on the website for citizens to decide what citizens care to believe or understand. I simply care to inform citizens of facts about how our government operates its vaccine programs and twists our vaccine laws, and you can decide what actions are best for you and your family, which in light of the current pandemic, may be an action which could lead to harm to you or your family. Vaccines do cause serious adverse vaccine-related injuries, and that statement is 100% correct.

Science must be proven with facts not by a single party or a small group of designated authorities endorsed by our government, but by citizens. And likewise, our laws must be informative for our citizens to understand what the consequences of any choice they make could be. Do citizens really understand they have limited legal rights and protections under the Vaccine Law? Do citizens care? Or would citizens prefer someone else make these choices for them? I prefer to make my choices for myself based on facts. Facts understood and discovered in science and shared among medical professionals and citizens.

CHAPTER 5

The Vaccine Information Statement

If you have had a vaccine, you have likely seen a Vaccine Information Statement (or commonly called a VIS) supplied by the national Centers for Disease Control and Prevention (also known as the CDC). And just for personal reference please make note, Safety is not in the CDC's name, just Control and Prevention. Safety is a wider concern suggested as collectively addressed by the CDC, FDA, NIH and ACIP for vaccines, which are Department of Health and Human Services (HHS) agencies and part of the Presidential Executive Branch policy team. Drug safety, specifically, generally falls to the FDA, as our nation's sole drug regulator. All medical professionals also have a required professional duty to address medical and drug concerns and must address both usage efficacy and adverse safety concerns for all drug and medical treatment options.

I display here a CDC Vaccine Information Statement for a group of vaccines known as Influenza (Flu) vaccines. The flu vaccine is formulated by scientists from a mix of viral influenza strains, which are inactivated or use a recombinant DNA (replication) process to create a flu-like antigen. The antigens are isolated using pharmaceutical methods to produce a vaccine containing inactive antigens in hopes that such antigens will trigger production of antibodies and an immune response which hopefully will provide protective immunity against specific stains of flu. The flu shot does not cover all influenza types, just the strains forecast to be circulating in a particular window of time.

If you have an interest in reviewing any other Vaccine Information Statement, all VISs are available from the CDC at: https://www.cdc.gov/vaccines/hcp/vis/current-vis.html. All health care providers are required by federal law to provide a Vaccine Information Statement to all patients receiving a vaccine (administered in whole or in parts) for diphtheria, tetanus, pertussis, measles, mumps, rubella, polio, hepatitis A, hepatitis B, Haemophilus influenzae type b (Hib), influenza, pneumococcal conjugate, meningococcal, rotavirus, human papillomavirus (HPV), or varicella (chickenpox). These Vaccine Information Statements must be provided by the vaccinating professional before each vaccine dose is administered. I emphasize the importance here not because it is the federal law, but because I have seen the law dismissed often as unimportant to many health care providers. A VIS is available online for all vaccines, but the Vaccine Act requires the VIS be presented as a point of starting a discussion for patients and providers. An actual dialog starter for patients to ask questions. Consider the VIS your opportunity to start asking questions and demanding further facts and details on vaccine SAFETY before you grant INFORMED CONSENT to be vaccinated, and please do not accept preprinted media pamphlets or promotional posters transferring the questions back to CDC statements. A medical professional should always answer your questions both directly and honestly about vaccine drug facts and vaccine literature to support answers to vital vaccine questions and concerns.

Influenza (Flu) Vaccine (Inactivated or Recombinant): *What you need to know*

Many Vaccine Information Statements are available in Spanish and other languages. See www.immunize.org/vis

Hojas de información sobre vacunas están disponibles en español y en muchos otros idiomas. Visite www.immunize.org/vis

1 Why get vaccinated?

Influenza vaccine can prevent **influenza (flu)**.

Flu is a contagious disease that spreads around the United States every year, usually between October and May. Anyone can get the flu, but it is more dangerous for some people. Infants and young children, people 65 years of age and older, pregnant women, and people with certain health conditions or a weakened immune system are at greatest risk of flu complications.

Pneumonia, bronchitis, sinus infections and ear infections are examples of flu-related complications. If you have a medical condition, such as heart disease, cancer or diabetes, flu can make it worse.

Flu can cause fever and chills, sore throat, muscle aches, fatigue, cough, headache, and runny or stuffy nose. Some people may have vomiting and diarrhea, though this is more common in children than adults.

Each year **thousands of people in the United States die from flu**, and many more are hospitalized. Flu vaccine prevents millions of illnesses and flu-related visits to the doctor each year.

2 Influenza vaccine

CDC recommends everyone 6 months of age and older get vaccinated every flu season. **Children 6 months through 8 years of age** may need 2 doses during a single flu season. **Everyone else** needs only 1 dose each flu season.

It takes about 2 weeks for protection to develop after vaccination.

There are many flu viruses, and they are always changing. Each year a new flu vaccine is made to protect against three or four viruses that are likely to cause disease in the upcoming flu season. Even when the vaccine doesn't exactly match these viruses, it may still provide some protection.

Influenza vaccine **does not cause flu**.

Influenza vaccine may be given at the same time as other vaccines.

3 Talk with your health care provider

Tell your vaccine provider if the person getting the vaccine:

- Has had an **allergic reaction after a previous dose of influenza vaccine**, or has any **severe, life-threatening allergies**.
- Has ever had **Guillain-Barré Syndrome** (also called GBS).

In some cases, your health care provider may decide to postpone influenza vaccination to a future visit.

People with minor illnesses, such as a cold, may be vaccinated. People who are moderately or severely ill should usually wait until they recover before getting influenza vaccine.

Your health care provider can give you more information.

CDC

U.S. Department of
Health and Human Services
Centers for Disease
Control and Prevention

4 Risks of a vaccine reaction

- Soreness, redness, and swelling where shot is given, fever, muscle aches, and headache can happen after influenza vaccine.
- There may be a very small increased risk of Guillain-Barré Syndrome (GBS) after inactivated influenza vaccine (the flu shot).

Young children who get the flu shot along with pneumococcal vaccine (PCV13), and/or DTaP vaccine at the same time might be slightly more likely to have a seizure caused by fever. Tell your health care provider if a child who is getting flu vaccine has ever had a seizure.

People sometimes faint after medical procedures, including vaccination. Tell your provider if you feel dizzy or have vision changes or ringing in the ears.

As with any medicine, there is a very remote chance of a vaccine causing a severe allergic reaction, other serious injury, or death.

5 What if there is a serious problem?

An allergic reaction could occur after the vaccinated person leaves the clinic. If you see signs of a severe allergic reaction (hives, swelling of the face and throat, difficulty breathing, a fast heartbeat, dizziness, or weakness), call **9-1-1** and get the person to the nearest hospital.

For other signs that concern you, call your health care provider.

Adverse reactions should be reported to the Vaccine Adverse Event Reporting System (VAERS). Your health care provider will usually file this report, or you can do it yourself. Visit the VAERS website at **www.vaers.hhs.gov** or call **1-800-822-7967**. *VAERS is only for reporting reactions, and VAERS staff do not give medical advice.*

6 The National Vaccine Injury Compensation Program

The National Vaccine Injury Compensation Program (VICP) is a federal program that was created to compensate people who may have been injured by certain vaccines. Visit the VICP website at **www.hrsa.gov/vaccinecompensation** or call **1-800-338-2382** to learn about the program and about filing a claim. There is a time limit to file a claim for compensation.

7 How can I learn more?

- Ask your healthcare provider.
- Call your local or state health department.
- Contact the Centers for Disease Control and Prevention (CDC):
  - Call **1-800-232-4636 (1-800-CDC-INFO)** or
  - Visit CDC's **www.cdc.gov/flu**

Vaccine Information Statement (Interim)
Inactivated Influenza Vaccine
8/15/2019 | 42 U.S.C. § 300aa-26

The Vaccine Act further mandates a medical record of each vaccine administered must be provided for the patient's permanent medical record. This record must be kept by the patient's primary care provider and/or the patient. A patient should also start keeping a copy of their medical records on file for review by any medical professional, and should regularly review the records for accuracy (for example did the doctor really advise you to do what the nurse put down in the record, and did the doctor sign-off on the nurse's or PA's notes). The more records kept on file the better. A brief, sloppy or encrypted note is of no use to medical professionals that try to make sense of poorly prepared medical records. Excellent medical records are a good first sign of an excellent medical practice. Patients should not just ask for good medical records but demand them, and demand a copy following every visit or at least annually, and if the medical professional is progressive, ask for full access to all medical records and medical notes online. As the patient, you own the medical record, and you should have full access to all medical records.

And before any professionals gets mad, understand poorly composed notes and poorly kept medical records will be harmful to any patient in any future litigation or medical review, as stupid lawyers and judges do not know how to read a medical notation or who said what to whom on which date and or even what treatments were authorized by which licensed professional, or maybe that is the point of why physicians keep poor records in the first place. For the record, only doctors and authorized doctor's agents can make a statement or recommend a medical treatment, and physicians must review and physically sign off on each recommendation for all patient recommended treatment plans. As many physicians are now merely supervising and treating from afar, with nurses and assistants acting as the face for the physician's care team. A nurse and an assistant have only limited treating authority restricted under state laws, not federal law. Under federal law, Courts are now okay with anyone on the medical team recording poor and false vaccine statements, if a record was presumably recorded by someone on the health care team, even if no physician signed off on records as required by law. A new change in federal court interpretations on who is responsible for a patient's health care services today, as it is no longer just the physician but the health care provider team that is responsible for a patient's care, and keep in mind vaccines are now held to a federal standard and not a state medical practice standard.

Under most state laws, the physician is the legal party all medical parties must report to for matters relating to a patient's treatment. Federal courts however have a different interpretation granting wider discretion, especially relating to vaccines. A VICP special master offering a legal opinion about vaccines that is nonsense is acceptable if the nonsense is kept in-house among a select group of federal judges. Again, federal drug supervision requirements do not match state requirements for vaccine record reporting requirements. Federal laws endorse less restrictive vaccine drug counseling and reporting requirements as noted in broad and relaxed terminology used in vaccine promotional literature.

Again, I strongly recommend patients keep both vaccine records and all medical records current. Ask your healthcare provider for a full medical records release form. These records should include any medical notes, which are legally part of the medical record, even the unprofessional comments made as side notes. If you start keeping records now, the costs should be minimal or free of charge. If you wait, the costs allowed under some state laws are ridiculous and an exploitation of patient rights for access to their own records. Add a lawyer to the mix and medical records can mysteriously go missing without a subpoena or court order. Records get lost, all the time. Let us start with these mandates, as both a VIS and medical record are mandated under both federal and state laws.

I say this as many health care providers fail the documentation and information requirements regularly. Sometimes failing upfront, sometimes in filing and recordkeeping, and often in retrieving and supplying accurate medical records. Patients have a right to this information, and it is mandatory they request medical records and information at the time of service. If printed, keep a file, or scan a copy into your computer. Do not expect your health care providers to keep good records for you, even as it is their job to do so.

I say request these documents for the patient's health, for without a correct medical record and without treatment information the patient is receiving substandard medical care. A trust relationship begins with every health care provider when medical services are started and with all follow-up services. Medical records and information given to patients are critical pieces to the medical decision-making process known as patient informed consent approval. Informed consent is the consent a patient gives to any health care provider to administer or deliver any medical drug or service.

Informed consent should be formalized as a signed consent granted by a patient but has often become informalized in today's medical practices. I suggest here, vaccines may often be administered without full patient informed consent and are often given under discretionary implied consent. A noted okay often means okay yes, not okay no. Doctors can make life or death medical decisions without consent, but vaccines are not life or death. I simply say all vaccinations require a medical informed consent by the patient, or patient's legal guardian. You may have seen these types of documents, as shown in a television show for example, but these documents are often poorly managed and awfully recorded in real-world practices. All patients should demand a copy of consent records be kept with a copy of their medical records.

Many health care workers are the worst in supplying documentation and even as technology has advanced, medical records are still incredibly poor. And without good medical records and recordkeeping, the quality and trust level for any medical professional judgement statement simply drops, as the information is uncertain and based on professional guesses and beliefs, rather than hard medical facts. On-the-fly best guess professional judgements by health care providers have become the norm, as government officials dilute the patient's rights and encourage on-the-fly medical decisions with limited information utilized for making informed consent decisions, which increases the risk of harm to patients.

Briefly, I list a few facts to review before getting a vaccine and requesting a vaccine record, a vaccine record must, by federal law, include:

- The vaccine manufacturer name. There are no generic vaccine manufacturers as vaccines are brand name only drugs.
- Lot number, each dose comes from a single lot relating to several thousand individual doses in various sized dosing bottles or individual doses. The lot number should be listed to certify the lot administered.

- Date of administration by an authorized health care provider. Ask for a copy of the vaccinating person's license certification to confirm the person is authorized to administer vaccines under state laws.
- Name, title, and business address of the health care professional administering the vaccine, as this may be different from the party keeping vaccine records.
- Name and title of the individual who administered the vaccine. Record professional license number and registration numbers of provider and prescriber, which is often different from a vaccination certification number.
- Date that the VIS is provided (and VIS publication date, which must be a current VIS).
- Site (e.g., deltoid area) and Route (e.g. intramuscular) of administration.
- Expiration date of the vaccine and certification of proper storage kept prior to administration.

These are simple written requirements for a vaccine record which must be issued to a patient and a patient's designated primary care physicians in all states. It is not optional, or at anyone's discretion, but a legal requirement. A patient should demand these records prior to vaccination, and with related medical records as required with any follow-up, including any documented vaccine reactions, which can be minor or serious, as the CDC suggests individuals are now responsible for reporting adverse reactions to the Vaccine Adverse Event Reporting System (VAERS) program.

I will suggest many medical professionals are only vaguely familiar with the VAERS program, and few have had direct contact with the program. The VAERS program is a "voluntary" reporting program, not a mandatory reporting program, and medical professionals can make such reports at their discretion, which is often never. Few medical professionals would voluntarily "volunteer" to do more work and report adverse vaccine events, unless they are serious about their job and are truly dedicated to their patients. Most reporting falls to insufficiently trained medical recordkeeping staff, who report whatever the physicians say must be reported, such as cause of death, or medical complication codes needed to get insurance authorization or payment. These would be the truly critical reports the doctors care most about, not a VAERS report.

If a patient genuinely wants to make sure a vaccine injury report is filed to VAERS, it would be best they file the report themself. It is not hard, and there is no standardized report form, but a bit of understanding of medical jargon would be helpful, as the VAERS information-taking representatives have only limited medical training. If you have a vaccine injury and can get your doctor to do this vital task, it would be valuable as they can supply clinical data, notes and values which a non-medical professional may not understand. The VAERS report however is a nonsensical practice in futility as a VAERS report is not a valid part of a vaccine injury claim but serve as a public display of mostly anonymous information used by government officials and researchers as a random collection of vaccine injury data. It is however proper to formally request your medical professional and health care providers that administered and/or prescribed the vaccine submit the VAERS report, and demand a copy of this report, as it would now be part of your medical record. In other words, you know, they know, and everyone will know you had a vaccine adverse reaction.

And if you file a vaccine injury claim, everyone can tie the two together, even where the records cloak privacy. Privacy laws will suggestively protect your information, but who needs privacy laws, as the special master and courts will openly discuss your injury with everyone in the public in their legal opinions. I suggest do not be shy, your medical privacy is not that big of a deal, or at least that is how it is with vaccines. The Health Insurance Portability and Accountability Act of 1996 (commonly referred to as HIPAA laws) have little meaning when it comes to vaccine matters, as such laws and rules are outdated and worthless in today's information technology driven world. I would even suggest the Vaccine Act is both out-of-date and out-of-synch in relationship to the present medical practices, but that is another problem our government has trouble with addressing, citizen privacy. Lack of personal privacy, I hate it, most citizens hate it, but our government sends to commercial and government interests to profit from and abuse our personal data and information. This is a problem our government can apparently never address, even as many other governments at least attempt to protect their citizens' privacy.

And back to the patient's informed consent statement, which is often loosely granted by patients verbally. All patients must understand many vaccines are administered under a broad prescription order known as a blanket prescription order. A pharmacist cannot normally authorize or prescribe a vaccine administration, and nurses or other trained vaccinating agents in a hospital are not always administering a vaccination under a primary care physician's order, although that may be the case in some instances. Most vaccines are administered under a blanket prescription order often by a physician who may have no prior knowledge or history of the patient. One of my primary reasons I do not vaccinate patients is I generally do not have access to any patient information to address a patient's health and medical concerns related to vaccines. Under these accepted practices, a medical professional is told to freely vaccinate patients and ask detailed questions later. If a patient does not mention any concerns, it is often assumed by the professional the answer to any concerns are none.

So, if all parties are blind, why should anyone care to address safety concerns. State laws often step in and mandate procedures and safety measures, but again vaccines fall primarily under federal law, not state laws. The only marginal risk a medical professional may have concerning vaccines are failing to follow a state mandated procedure, in which case the medical professional may get a hand slap, or if protected by corporate lawyers a private reprimand, often simply a shame, shame, shame on them for their poor practices.

And it is vital a parent understand they alone are the sole informed consent giver for their child, or acting as a legal guardian for individuals unable to give legal informed consent for themselves which is legally defined under state laws, not federal laws. If you are starting to get confused by how each action applies under state or federal law do not feel you are alone, as most attorneys also fail in understanding the many quirks of both state and federal vaccine drug and medical laws. The individual's rights to make informed choices are mandatory under all laws but often get mixed up in the discussion of law. And one way to always address discretionary laws is with lots and lots of records, and a statement of informed consent. If you make a bad choice, then you made a bad choice. If you made the bad choice for a child, then you made the bad choice for your child or loved one, but the government has an equally vital responsibility to give you all available information and facts to make these informed and educated choices. It is a dual responsibility, as it relates to the responsibilities of parents and our government.

I know this sounds like a lot of records for a single vaccine, but your government wants to make sure you are fully informed and in compliance with the Vaccine Act. Nobody tells patients this anymore, often like the failure to fully counsel patients when prescribing or dispensing a prescription drug or recommending an OTC medication without checking with the patient on medical and prescription histories. Doctors are legally liable, so the less information supplied the better for their practice. Often treating physicians and medical professionals make discretionary professional judgements based on limited information. Again, the VIS is a suggested discussion starter, so do not miss the opportunity to ask important vaccine safety questions.

At this point, it should be clear, the CDC Vaccine Information Statement is a conceptual legal information statement of little administrative or enforcement value in the real-world practice setting. The CDC Vaccine Information Statement should be a starting point for discussions and not an end of a discussion, such as handing the Vaccine Information Statement slip of paper to the patient as they are being prepared for a jab. This type of action is inappropriate as it is with all prescription drugs. Vaccines are a prescription drug and must be given the same respect as other prescription drugs, and even over-the-counter drugs. This however is often not the case, as vaccines are treated with broad discretion as a public safety tool rather than being noted as a dangerous drug. Citizens should demand vaccinating professionals provide the same information and full list of risks as can be requested for any prescription drug. Professional oversight and counseling are a professional legal requirement, but few parties follow the rules or law, as enforcement of vaccine safety protocols are often discretionary. How do multiple heads of local and federal agencies claim discretionary authority over vaccines? That is an interesting question, but an answer few agency leaders care to lay claim to other than an implied shared public health interest. Vaccine promotional advocacy statements are more important than vaccine safety concerns to most government agency leaders.

Again, vaccines are often administered at a patient's request under a blanket prescription order. The patient is briefly counseled but the patient alone often must determine a suggestive balance of risks to benefits as being an appropriate balance in their personal analysis of risks relative to benefits of being vaccinated. All vaccine risks and safety concerns are not fully addressed in the CDC's Vaccine Information Statements. Administering a vaccine is not a particularly difficult task, and our government has reduced the vaccination process to being an exceptionally simple "robotic-like" task almost anyone can do, which requires little drug counselling or vital safety information be given to a patient. I simply ask patients to learn about informed consent, if you do not recall what an informed consent is, then demand facts and information which will allow you to make such informed decisions regarding a vaccine. As a pharmacist, I would be happy to help patients be informed citizens and to be vaccinated as informed citizens, as that is the citizen's rightful choice to make. I would simply prefer citizens be informed of all vaccine drug safety concerns and benefits, which the CDC does not supply in its VIS but can be found in multiple medical resources.

Our government often suggests their agencies are the best, if not sole, source of valuable vaccine information, but most countries do not outsource manufacturing regulation and surveillance of vaccine safety concerns to multiple agencies. Or even allow outside vaccines from global manufacturers to enter the domestic market, without extensive oversight. Our government funds a huge vaccine operation but runs it as if they alone independently determine which vaccines are best for all citizens through oversight by federal agencies. Our government portrays itself as the leader of global healthcare, which while being an honorable goal is far from a realistic statement of our government's practices.

Our government relies on a loosely tied regulatory administrative safety model to suggest regulation of vaccines and many drugs. Other nations look to our healthcare business model as an example of what not to do for citizen safety and protection, as few countries attempt to work under the same healthcare busines model as our government offers as the "world's best" model for healthcare. Our capitalist health business model often does not protect our citizens, and often overcharges consumers for important products and services. Other countries look at our health care system as a failing outdated capitalist system, but are happy to contribute to its downfall, or profit from the business model's weaknesses which are numerous. Many countries have better vaccine reporting systems which discuss and address vaccine protocol safety and efficacy in more open forums.

A review of the CDC's Vaccine Information Statement for context and usefulness to all citizens is called for as reasonable. I present the influenza VIS as a reference; as all Vaccine Information Statements are more or less the same. A COVID-19 Vaccine Information Statement will most likely be similar to the influenza VIS but will likely only list a few adverse side effects as part of its safety profile as many adverse vaccine reactions will not be current or reported from limited clinical studies, but what happens with an influenza vaccine, a viral based vaccine, would also generally apply to a COVID-19 vaccine.

I suggest a review of the influenza VIS should provide citizens with a generalized understanding of both the influenza (flu) vaccine and the upcoming COVID-19 vaccine. The understood risks and benefits will likely be similar and should be addressed using the same practices for evaluating and making an informed consent decision, or at least until further information and data is collected. Vaccine safety for any vaccine should not be assumed by citizens. Safety should be documented and demanded by citizens as based on reported clinical case reports and drug studies. The CDC states our government does this. I say with conviction both the CDC and FDA do not fully address all vaccine safety concerns unless demanded to do so by citizens.

When you review a Vaccine Information Statement, consider the VIS a brief informational statements: The CDC always begins a Vaccine Information Statement with the listed vaccine often grouped, such as in my example an influenza (flu) vaccine, which broadly covers all influenza-type vaccines. There are four different types of influenza viruses: influenza A, B, C, and D. Influenza A and B are the only types of influenza that cause widespread infections in humans. Type A and C Influenza can also cause infections in other animal species such as birds, dogs, and pigs. Major human infectious outbreaks of influenza are associated with influenza virus types A and/or B. Type A and B viral strains are used to formulate the mixture for annual flu vaccine formulations every year. Type C influenza viruses are also quite common and are related to viral strains that cause infections and reactions leading to simple cold symptoms and upper respiratory and/or nasal complications and may not require any medical treatment beyond rest, fluids and treatment of symptoms. All influenza virus types are considered highly contagious and in general cause similar illness and symptoms in varying degrees. There is currently no cure for an influenza viral infection. An antiviral drug treatment is as close as one can get to a curative treatment. A vaccine is not a cure and is only preventative if the vaccine antigen matches the circulating virus being spread between sick patients throughout a population. In recent years, flu vaccines have had a range of effectiveness in the 40 - 60% range, in good years. Antiviral medications are effective in managing many influenza strains but are not considered a fully effective cure. If you get sick from a flu virus, your body will go through a process of developing antibodies under natural immunity, which will still occur with antiviral drugs. Antivirals often only shorten the length of time a patient is sick from the flu virus.

Antiviral medications are best to use early in the onset of the infection cycle, and will shorten the viral infection, but does not kill the virus. Antivirals act more like some antibiotics that slow down the process of pathogen growth and give the patient's body a chance to respond to the viral threat rather than outright killing the virus, by interfering with the virus's replication processes. If timed right, an antiviral is a beneficial and useful drug, if the prescribed antiviral works on the specific virus strain being treated. However, there can also be poor matches of antivirals to treatable viral type infections and antivirals that miss the mark when addressed by poorly trained prescribers. If a doctor is guessing and is wrong, the antiviral option can be less useful than one would hope, and antivirals also have risks of adverse reactions, which are often well-documented and given to patients to review and evaluate before accepting as a treatment option. Many cases of influenza can be treated with simple drug protocols and rest which can help the body fight the flu infection and develop natural immunity. The adage "Feed a cold (a viral infection) and starve a fever (often a higher fever in a bacterial infection)" is an old saying that has been around for centuries, which is partly true. Like many infectious treatment plans, the idea originated during the Middle Ages when people first observed there were two kinds of illnesses, those with a fever, and those without. The illnesses caused by low temperatures, such as a cold, needed to be fueled, so eating was recommended. And the fever needs to go through "the sweats" to sweat out the disease in bacterial infections. But understand doctors were not so scientific back then, just observers and speculators. Both bacterial and viral infection-types are fought off with good nutrition and fluids, so rest and hydrate as the body permits. Recent studies have shown eating helps the body recover in viral flu-like cases; and glucose-based diets may help in bacterial infectious cases but are not as helpful with added proteins and fats which may make the bacterial infections worse. If applied properly a good nutritional plan is important to restoring the body back to good health.

Inflammation is also often a big complication of infectious diseases which often leads to a secondary or even tertiary infection. Addressing the inflammation can help reduce medical complications. This process involves multiple organs of the endocrine system, primarily served by the adrenal glands of the kidney which make natural steroids. Proper dosing of supplementary corticosteroid (for example prednisone) medication is useful in calming all inflamed tissue and can often reduce inflammation linked to infections by 30% or more. If treated and administered properly, corticosteroids can significantly shorten the length of an infectious illness. As corticosteroids are aiding the immune system in a period of crisis and transition, or again commonly called finding balance. Steroids are nonspecific and calms all inflamed body tissues but can be tricky to administer. Again, vaccines do not help the body find homeostatic balance, but helps the body develop antibodies through a protective immune mechanism; but such protection also has a cost, and that cost can be an unfound liability and risk of medical complications, which is a common complication related to all drugs, just operating under different mechanisms of action and injury. Again, vaccine-related injuries are poorly reported, but has often been tied to inflammation and immune-system-mediated factors.

I mention here, COVID-19 is thought to currently have two strains (or perhaps more strains) of the coronavirus in circulation around the world. The strain affecting the U.S. population has been noted as being highly contagious, but perhaps not as impactful on the immune system as the original strain found in China. This is however in an early stage of detection and is not fully certain, as the determination of whether we are seeking protection from one or several strains of COVID-19 is currently uncertain and mostly speculative. A lot like the guessing that goes on with influenza vaccines when it comes time to develop a formulation months before the flu vaccines are made and distributed. Are we searching for a vaccine that hits one, two or more viral strains? And could the strains change and evolve over time like many other viruses? These are critical questions, but not as serious to all citizens today as the infectious disease only affects certain individuals, often with serious comorbidities that impact medical complications. COVID-19 and influenza are both viral infections. They are not the same types of viruses which are caused by different virus classes (or grouping classifications). COVID-19 is a coronavirus, not an influenza class virus. Both viruses can lead to a highly contagious respiratory infection which can lead to respiratory complications and secondary infections. Secondary infections are often more complicated bacterial or fungal infections, which further complicate the medical state of illness or pre-existing medical conditions. Life and health in general become harder to address when a patient develops a viral or bacterial infection.

All viral strains are isolated as originating from a specific group of host species. Novel viral infections often change in structure as a method of adapting and as related to adjusting to the host and the host's living environment. These adaptions can occur quickly, depending on the viral types and complexity of adaption. Viral adaption and changes are part of the problem with viral based vaccinations. Which asks the question, who can work faster and more efficiently as adapters to change, viruses or scientists? Unfortunately, even as the science and viral behaviors are understood, keeping up with viral infections and adaptions are often a challenging task. And keeping up with medical complications related to vaccines, especial viral-based vaccines, often takes years, if not decades to address, as the vaccine formulation is constantly changing and shifting. Influenza and COVID-19 vaccines should be considered to have less documented safety profiles, due to poorly reported adverse drug reactions not being formally explained with changing formulations administered each year. Gaps in safety data are commonly bridged from year to year to form a guesstimate for a vaccine safety profile. Pharmacovigilant post-approval studies and reporting to the FDA for year-specific and formulation-specific vaccine related injuries often takes years to decades to analyze reported cases and data. This type of random regulatory reporting and analysis of adverse vaccine reactions is speculative and is not an entirely safe drug evaluation practice. As many serious vaccine injuries are often ignored and not addressed in a continuing safe evaluation practice, as required under normal drug reporting requirements mandated under routine drug laws.

A competing testing analysis problem also develops in isolating and reporting these changes and viral adaptions. As shifts in how the disease spreads through human-to-human contact, human-to-animal contract, surfaces-to-human contact, airborne contact, or even insect-to-human contact in some viral infections. Speculation often leads to years of analysis, but often the full mechanisms of spread are never fully figured out. A virus can pass through various host transmission mechanisms which are not discovered for years. If mechanisms of spread are isolated, this is considered good when compared to past infectious outbreaks like the Black Plague outbreaks which took many centuries to discover its likely source was bacteria carried by fleas on rats and mice. Better sanitation and controlling the rodent population dramatically changed the levels of infections. Influenza and COVID-19 viruses are noted as being highly contagious and appears to spread via human-to-human and human-to-animal contacts, with added spread from surface and short-distance airborne contacts. Masks, protective gear, and goggles/shields may be useful or completely worthless depending on various sources of transmission and a likelihood of exposure from multiple sources. More specialized protective gear is protective in a closed environment but may have insignificant impact in preventing the long-term spread in an open public environment. This is not an argument for or against citizens wearing any protective gear, as it certainly does not hurt to add protective gear as a tool in limiting the spread, but likely does not halt the eventual spread to most citizens over a longer period. The original recommended protection suggested by the CDC and medical professionals initially as a guideline, which was the general statement that all citizens do not need to wear masks is largely accurate but broader use of protective equipment and masks by the public will "slow" the spread. Some scientists guessing the virus may "die-out" on its own. The cycle of spread and longevity of most viral infections are largely unknown, as infectious outbreaks could be a short-term event, an annual event or an ongoing infectious disease with many irregular distribution patterns covering many centuries. COVID-19 infections will impact most, if not all, citizens in some fashion, and when and how it changes over time is a speculative complex medical concern.

Our government authorities love to think they can control or regulate naturally occurring infectious diseases in some manner. As government agencies have tried to guess and control naturally occurring infections for centuries. Our government dedicates enormous resources to be at the forefront of infectious disease control, and often takes the steps it believes will be the answer to controlling outbreaks, but the answers by authorities are generally speculative. Which leads to the question, are authorities better at answering concerns of infectious diseases with speculative answers, or can citizens address these concerns on their own, if given proper guidance and a complete list of potential risks, including vaccine injuries? The constitutional answer is the individual must be given facts by authorities when they are known and should issue best practices when they are understood. Speculative nonsensical decisions and recommendations by authorities are useless to citizens but are often passed along as being superior in particulars in some manner. For example, ignoring an adverse vaccine reaction which is rare in occurrence does not make the vaccine injury not real. The adverse injury problem can get worse, and in many instances have gotten worse as the science behind the drug reaction are ignored and can and will lead to further adverse drug reactions in a greater number of individuals, involving a greater number of drugs. Passive inert actions do not solve serious drug problems.

So, I go back to the influenza VIS, where Influenza vaccine manufacturers develop flu vaccines that are either monovalent, trivalent, or currently a quadrivalent influenza vaccines in the United States. Meaning the vaccine has either 1, 3, or 4 types of virus antigens present in each formulation. This formulation mixture is predetermined months in advance before manufacturing begins and is generally based on differing circulating types in the Northern and Southern Hemispheres, as agreed upon in partnership with the World Health Organization (WHO). So, the current influenza vaccine shot is in fact 1, 3 or 4 vaccines wrapped into one shot. COVID-19 may also be more than one strain, but as it is currently being tested as a single strain, which may only target the most likely circulating strain in the U.S. and may not cover all strains circulating globally. Speculative science often misses its target. An inaccurate viral vaccine formulation mix is often manufactured and distributed during many flu seasons. COVID may similarly be off-target and ineffective, initially being found as effective then becoming less effective during subsequent future outbreaks.

Many other countries are also creating a COVID-19 vaccine for the virus type found specifically in their region, as many countries produce their own influenza vaccine formulation based on their own scientists' speculative guesses to circulating viral types. How the virus evolves is hard to predict, as the virus may shift differently in different regions. A single universal global-based vaccine for COVID-19 is unlikely to be developed under the current global vaccine development system. It is uncertain whether COVID-19 will be short or long-term in causing infectious outbreaks. Or if a more problematic virus or bacteria will come alongside COVID, Influenza, Pneumonia, or other infectious diseases, and cause further widespread medical crises. Government actions should be preemptive in making infectious disease preparations. Speculation on top of speculation is not an answer to addressing many medical and infectious concerns for protection, treatment, and addressing adverse risks related to the vaccine.

It should be highlighted that vaccines are not always the answer for all infectious diseases, as influenza vaccines have consistently been unsuccessful in addressing most influenza outbreaks for over a century. Some doctors freely speculate injections of all vaccinations are the best and only protective treatment plan for infectious diseases, by suggesting all vaccines will "activate" the immune system, suggesting the immune system response to developing immunity is like pushing the power button to start a machine. Just start the machine and go, which is not how it works in the immune system. Many doctors and authorities often suggest all vaccines supply some theoretical relief and protection. This concept however is mostly false as an increased immune system activity does not automatically lead to the development of the right antibodies needed for protection. These practices of pushing vaccines to everyone often simply leads to a false sense of security which will not affect the virus or bacteria targeted as lacking antibodies needing to be developed by the immune system for protective immunity. While doctors will suggest some theoretical net gain in immunity if given all available vaccines, the negative aspects of heightened immune system activity which include concerns that lead to serious vaccine-related injuries are often marginalized in an otherwise promotional argument pushing the protective benefits of vaccines. In short, vaccine-related injuries are noted as secondary concerns and are regularly marginalized as serious concerns.

The CDC Vaccine Information Statement is a thin and general legal document designed to address a narrow subject matter in the easiest discussion format possible. The VIS does not demand a need to discuss vaccine injuries or even the vaccine's relative effectiveness. Alternative treatment protocols are left off the VIS as this is a noted promotional-type informational statement. If you want to learn more about vaccine-related injuries, you will likely need to do so on your own, as the government is not doing their job to help citizens. And if our government does not know or care to inform citizens, many medical professionals also do not have the answers to develop safe treatment protocols. The Vaccine Information Statements are not designed to provide you more detailed facts, or even point patients to professional manufacturer product information statements, and other public vaccine drug safety-related documents which may be difficult to find but are available through public resources.

Doctors and pharmacists have access to these vaccine medical literature reports, but not all literature is readily available as academic researchers often limit access to research and recently discovered science, but will often grant access to medical professionals. The profit-driven angle to pharmaceutical and medical research often slows down the discoveries and application of therapies used to treat vaccine-related injuries, as research funding is limited, and peer review of findings can take years or even decades. Government-assisted funding for research is often limited and discretional, and vaccine injury causational analysis by any party of the government is almost nonexistent or not in public circulation.

Again, hiding facts and keeping decision-making choices in-house among authorities, not given to citizens to discuss for best treatment options which is an exceedingly poor regulatory practice for our government to have as a standard practice, with discretionary judgements made relating to level of importance often made in the name of their value to public health. And asking a legal professional or special master to understand the mechanisms of a vaccine injury, forget about it. Until a panel of experts can sit down and put it in a book specifically written for the HHS authorities to read, vaccine injuries are not addressed, and even as the injury may be noted in medical literature, it will take decades to reach a VICP special master, who simply does not and probably should not attempt to evaluate the science themselves. Science facts and opinions by nonscientists will often clash in terms of their relative value to individual citizens verse the larger general population, but hopefully in a small collision, and hopefully those small collisions do not result in a serious medical complication for you and your loved ones.

Be prepared before you vaccinate and prepare to ask as many questions as you like when you talk to a licensed vaccinating medical professional. The vaccinating medical professional should be fully trained to administer and to address all vaccine usage and safety concerns. But use caution when using unlicensed "government-designated" healthcare providers our government assigns as being acceptably trained vaccinators to rapidly distribute and administer a vaccine with limited testing done in a short window of time. As this would be a military styled operation with few individual freedoms or protections concerning drug and vaccine procedural safety problems. You should feel comfortable in the vaccine-related answers you receive from medical professionals and be comfortable with any adverse vaccine risk concerns discussed, and the possibility the medical professionals may share additional conflicting concerns which should be understood and highlighted as specific concerns related to a patient's current or recent medical condition.

An FDA Freedom of Information Act (FOIA) information requests may also be a good source of additional drug facts and more widely-reported vaccine injuries often marked confidential by manufacturers when reported to the FDA, which is required data but not easily accessible to the public. To access such information, simply search for how to make a FOIA request at the FDA.gov website. FOIA requests for drug information should list specific questions and use medical terminology related to drugs and medical complications whenever possible. Perhaps you have a specific medical condition, so you would request "all post-marketing and pharmacovigilant data and reports for a specific date range for medical condition X, as it relates to vaccine(s) manufactured under the Brand Names X by vaccine manufacturer X". It is always best to know your medical condition and related terms.

And demand a quick response but be prepared for a long wait for an answer. Six months is a reasonable wait period. Two years or more is a normal wait period according to the FDA's top FOIA request officials. Doctors and medical professionals have similar long waits, so do not feel disheartened. The FDA, like every federal agency, will claim to be understaffed and have limited resources. Just remember the same staff and resources are approving and authorizing drugs and vaccines for all citizens, and often fail to ensure all drugs maintain and report drug safety concerns post-approval to all parties in a proper legally required fashion, including vaccines which have a specialized group of FDA staff dedicated just to vaccine safety and effectiveness. I can point you to their office and phone numbers if you care to discuss any specific concerns, some are friendly but not fully knowledgeable on all vaccine facts. A scary thought but a real concern in the real world of drug regulation and pharmaceutical oversight.

In general, doctors are a good source for general vaccine questions. A doctor who is a specialist may also be a better source for specialized medical questions related to a specific medical conditions or risks, but such specialists are not always the best drug experts outside of their specialized drug regimens they prescribe regularly. Many doctors, even specialists, often do not read a drug manufacturer's product information statements which lists drug adverse effects, warnings, and precautions. I have had doctors on many occasions suggesting the manufacturer product information (PI) statement is misleading or inaccurate, stating the PI has limited or no studies to support the facts the PI states as understood. It is often a weird medical discussion, when a pharmacist and doctor communicate on drug safety issues, as the doctors are often simply trying to understand how a drug will work and which patients will see the most benefit, but rarely learn many of the medial complications and drug actions and mechanisms of actions as applied to a drug throughout the body.

Let us just say doctors are a lot like government authorities, and make a "good faith" effort but not always their "best" effort, and believe their job is to address the clinical medical treatment plan and sometimes believe a new pharmaceutical drug with a less developed safety record may offer a better treatment plan to patients, or at least that is what they were told by the cute drug marketing representatives pushing the newer high-cost pharmaceutical drugs at the resort/spa. Some adverse drug reaction warnings take years to be addressed and listed on the manufacturer's product information statements. Citizens should understand after graduating from school most doctors will only retain 10% of what they were taught, and retained knowledge decreases every year, unless an individual aggressively pursues knowledge which is relevant and applicable to their areas of practice and interest.

Vaccines plummet as an area of interest in this huge vacuum of medical and drug knowledge. Many medical professionals have not engaged in aggressive pursuit of vaccine drug information as they simply try to manage their day-to-day tasks and duties, which is simply called trying to make a living which is increasingly harder to do. If an authority says there is a need to vaccinate everyone, many medical professionals just accept the recommendation and attempt to vaccinate everyone as a professional duty and in some cases to keep their jobs. Believe it or not, many health care companies mandate vaccination practices regardless of a professional's training or specialty, with implied threats to either vaccinate patients or else.

Vaccine science arguments are complex for sure, as many parties do not follow the drug science and facts, but common vaccine scientific facts are accessible, although sometimes made more difficult to access by vaccine manufacturers. The manufacturer's full disclosure drug Product Information statement (also known as a PI statement) is in general a complete statement of the most recognized and suspected adverse vaccine risks accepted as understood adverse events for a given drug. Doctors often have these in their office as an outdated (not current) collection of PI statements in a reference called a Physician's Desk Reference (or PDR) which is an abbreviated and incomplete PI collection of drug data. The full drug profile in a PI is reviewed by hundreds or thousands of experts in medicine and in the pharmaceutical field. The FDA requires many, many experts to review the data and facts statements before approving such product information statements for publication by the manufacturer. The FDA approves PI statements but is not the publisher. The FDA and manufacturer however do make PI statements available online to the public.

What the manufacturers do not always make available in the PI statement are medical complications listed as suspected or likely adverse drug reactions (or ADRs), which are often discovered but simply go into a basket of more likely or highly suspected adverse reactions most likely thought to be related to the drug and offer the reported ADRs for the FDA to consider as possible additions to the PI statement. This basket of suspected ADRs are then handed out and evaluated by many experts. The time taken to evaluate an ADR however is often very slow, with normal drugs taking in the area of 20 years to address some drug injury concerns, and thanks to the Vaccine Act and VICP with its newfangled roadblocks, one can possibly see an ADR added to a vaccine PI in 40 to 50 years, not exactly a warp speed path to scientific safety discoveries. But who is keeping track? Not our government.

And certainly not for the injured individuals discarded by our government as insignificant as relating to the public health needs of the masses. Imagine, a drug is approved by the FDA, when a serious adverse drug-related event is discovered and documented, and 20 years later the FDA slowly gets around to issuing an Important Safety Information (an ISI) Warning, which is then added to the PI as a Boxed Warning (in other industries they may call such warnings a red sticker buyer beware warning), which does not mean the drug cannot be used, it just means citizens and medical professionals have been warned about serious adverse drug risks, where such information must be shared with a patient.

But there is no need to imagine this, as this is what really happens in our government. And in prior individual cases where injuries happened in the years before the official government warning was issued. But that sort of problem is left to be worked out by manufacturers and lawyers, except wait with vaccines the problem is left to be worked out by our government and the lawyers. The vaccine manufacturers are out of the vaccine liability picture. Manufacturers will not take action to address a prior undisclosed suspected but known adverse drug reaction injury without a lawsuit, and lawyers will not usually take on a lawsuit unless it is a class action lawsuit. Sorry lawyers, no class action lawsuits available in the vaccine drug class. The Vaccine Act axed that little legal maneuver. Citizens should be concerned with vaccine safety information as reduced vaccine liability to all vaccine parties makes the need for quicker action and documentation of adverse vaccine-related injuries critical to fulfilling the individual's need in becoming informed citizens, and working with informed medical professionals who have a duty to provide accurate data and information to citizens. The FDA and our government routinely neglect fulfilling their duties to provide these vital resources for discussion among all parties interested in vaccine safety concerns.

Why does the FDA slow down the evaluation process or not force further swift research and vigilance after the drug's first approval is granted by the FDA commissioner? That could be a good question for many authorities to answer, but often the FDA, or simply the FDA commissioner is satisfied with data and grants approval or the commissioner can also at any time ban a drug or drug class that impacts even a small orphan population also at the commissioner's discretion. It is a discretionary action granted as an authoritative action to the commissioner, and any drug concern could drag out for years and give little data to be shared with the public, except for the highly curious citizens that demand facts found in secret marked "confidential" reports that are found through targeted FOIA requests. This of course gets into the area of liability, and where the manufacturer has interests in managing the risks, while making a profit to cover years of research and development costs, and the FDA lets the drug manufacturers and doctors develop a more well-rounded safety profile, which could be very bad, or maybe in time better understood and managed. A sort of double-edged sword issue which vaccine products in particular have lived with for centuries. Most citizens simply blindly accept the poor discussions of safety relating to drug-induced injuries and do not know how to address the government's poor efforts to address drug safety concerns for all citizens. That is a concern I will discuss in more detail later in the book.

Keep in mind many government actions are discretionary actions (for example, could our government even open for business each day without a discretionary Presidential executive order), and many discretionary actions often lead to harmful misfortunes for many citizens. Influenza and coronaviruses are viral infections that can change over time. For this reason, vaccine reported data is less reliable and judgements are often based on prior years' data, which may be older vaccine data not specific to the currently used vaccine formulation. A novel vaccine generally has extremely limited data, and often refers to older data as a source for current projections and speculative projections as the FDA and manufacturers cannot collect data fast enough to be confirmed as accurate. This speculative and questionable data is the highest cause for concerns relating to adverse drug risk reporting.

As the FDA's vaccine safety staff often do not attempt to address smaller, less-certain vaccine adverse events discovered in patients, but prefer to watch for many more obvious adverse concerns over an extended period, and draw a theoretical discretionary line as they see fit, not as citizens may see fit in a real life evaluation of vaccine-related adverse events. Could this hurt a child? Sorry but the FDA and experts may not understand a concern, or the concerns may not be fully researched by our government right now. Maybe the "experts" can figure out the ADR or get to the concern in a few decades, which is what it sounds a lot like when citizens talk to FDA officials and the FDA commissioner's office. There are paths to resolution of any adverse vaccine-related reaction, but again the government's administrative paths are exceptionally long, and the process may skip over many injured parties before being addressed.

This does not suggest the FDA will deny a vaccine injury has been occurring in a specific population, but simply means they will not be addressing the concern quickly as a matter of discretion. The discriminatory blend of medicine, science, and law all use discretion, and require citizens blindly accept limited access to facts. The current influenza Vaccine Information Statement notes GBS is now an understood and accepted risk related to the flu vaccine. This flu vaccine-induced neurological complication has been understood for decades, going back to 1976. The HHS and FDA took 35 years to investigate and agree with the original findings of several prominent scientists. And another 6 years, from 2012 to 2018, to add the adverse injury to the VICP Injury Table, and another year to add it to the Influenza Vaccine Information Statement. One could argue why even bother, as it is such a rare adverse event, but perhaps the government felt compelled to add it to the VIS as a legal disclosure rather than seek out actual injured patients. If you believe our government addresses these vaccine ADR concerns promptly upon learning about the serious adverse injury, you are either gullible or an unconcerned citizen, which could one day impact your life. Again, do not miss the window to file a GBS or SIRVA claim for vaccine-related injuries or you may miss out and get nothing.

I do not suggest the FDA is the sole party seeking understanding of adverse vaccine-induced reaction discoveries, but the FDA works with many other parties who work under an umbrella of confidentiality and liability protection, as many vaccine parties often share responsibility in protecting each other. Manufacturers who market vaccines in the U.S. surely do their part to conceal adverse vaccine-induced event reports, as many simply do not submit all information to the FDA, which can often be reported and published in other countries' regulatory drug agencies years before the FDA will act on the reported injuries. Such information can put an adverse risk in a state of conflict within multiple agencies for years, if not decades. A false claim of transparency by our federal agencies about vaccines facts often leads to misreported or unreported vaccine-induced safety concerns which can lead to harm to many citizens.

I have come across many profit and promotion-driven medical and healthcare practices marketed to the public many times in my professional life which are stated as having benefits to the public but offer little real value to patients. Some schemes with interesting tie-ins to government and public officials that should have been addressed by the regulatory officials with oversight of the concerns but instead authorities let the concerns grow bigger, as many schemes have government officials with financial ties that benefited from the scheme. The required accountability and public transparency to private and even government schemes are in general extremely poor. Our government has done little to improve healthcare transparency and addressing adverse drug injury concerns for citizens. These types of uncaring and unthoughtful acts must at some point, be rejected by citizens.

The CDC Vaccine Information Statement is not a science-driven consumer information statement, but a promotion-driven consumer vaccine marketing statement. Pharmacies already provide you with more information than the CDC does with basis computer software printout about all drugs, including vaccines. The VIS supplies a lot of information which is outdated and driven by legal requirements, as mandated by the Vaccine Act. And not valuable medical information the public and medical professionals mandate as necessary for supplying information to citizens for informed consent discussions.

A pharmacist Vaccine Information Statement would let you know exactly what vaccine you are taking, what the dose and route of administration is, who the manufacturer is, what types of viral strains are in the vaccine. A pharmacist VIS would cover not only notable benefits and suggested effectiveness but would also state what prior year efficacy and current expected efficacies for the current vaccine are as stated from current vaccine studies. A vaccine that has a 40% or less rate of effectiveness (my personal standards are a little higher than this) may suggest an obvious reason to reject a vaccine. And a pharmacist VIS would provide a complete list of known and suspected vaccine injuries, including those with unknown causational linkage. Reporting of ALL known and suspected vaccine-related injuries should be mandatory as a required duty of the vaccinating professional regardless of the professional's understanding of the underlying risk. And it is reasonable copies of any report of a vaccine-related ADR with details of the ADR must be provided to the injured party at a patient's request, and not submitted voluntarily at the medical professional's personal discretion, which is often never, which is currently the professional standard. A required follow-up of any suspected or known adverse drug reaction should also be mandatory and required as a reported injury to VAERS and the VICP. Professional indifference and poorly reported ADRs are the biggest problem with furthering the need to properly address adverse vaccine-related injuries. Again, poor pharmacovigilant reporting does not fully address the vaccine safety and liability concerns but makes these concerns more muddied and discretionary for all parties. Citizens have a right to use discretion in evaluating and judging facts before making informed consent decisions. Government authorities try to take away this right for citizen discretion by using their own discretions as authoritative rules and laws.

In a pharmacist VIS, the VAERS reporting system would be replaced by a valid system for reporting research data and vaccine facts, with mandatory follow-up recordings and easier access to reported data for all citizens. And the Vaccine Injury Compensation Program, the VICP is a falsely developed legal program that suggests a citizen safety net exists which in reality is neither honest nor true. Any medical professional that would devote any time to investigate the VICP program could easily come to the same conclusion. Doctors and pharmacists often fail to understand the VICP program's focus as the Vaccine Law is not a priority in understanding laws which apply to their practice. Medical schools briefly instruct medical professionals about the Vaccine Act, and foreign-trained doctors have even less required knowledge about our drug and vaccine laws. And the vaccine laws and vaccine legal processes are rarely asked as questions as a part of any professional medical licensure testing, certification, or continuing education requirements to continue practicing as a licensed medical professional. Higher educational standards and understanding of vaccine laws should be mandatory and should be required for all medical professionals that even bring up the subject of vaccines. Let us start by making vaccine education and vaccine information a widely understood subject matter with needed understanding of both vaccine actions and more importantly safety concerns.

I hope my professional review of a VIS will serve the public in making their own informed consent decisions based on understood vaccine facts and evidence, not broad promotional claims that have little value to individuals who can be harmed by vaccines. Should you choose to accept the CDC recommended guidelines, and condensed FDA data, it is your choice. I am not here to stop any individual from receiving a vaccine they decide as being the right medical choice for themself, but I simply provide fair warning that vaccine drug information is poorly reported and addressed by Vaccine Inc. It is your responsibility to make yourself an informed citizen, and to demand more detailed vaccine information whenever you feel a need for more information or data, and you absolutely have a right to reject an offered vaccine that has been incompletely and unprofessionally addressed by our government or likely by the medical professional offering the vaccination service. The best advice I can offer is be informed and make good healthcare choices. There are medical professionals here to help.

CHAPTER 6

Do No Harm To A Child vs. The "So What" Argument

This an argument I feel strongly about, as a parent and as a medical professional. The highest level of concern relating to drugs are associated with children, as all drugs have a sperate set of usage guidelines and observed adverse precautions for children. Vaccines are no different from other drugs, yet vaccines often follow the same guidelines and reporting standards as noted for adults. Medical professionals fall into one of two groups. Those that follow their medical Oath and promise to do no harm, and those that believe the "so what" argument, as in "so what" if a child is harmed as the benefits of the drug are more important to protect the child and society than the harm which can be caused by the drug. The "so what" argument can also be set on a sliding rule. Where the risk can be low, or the risk can be high, and parties can use a sliding rule to justify a "so what".

In medical terminology, this is often called the professional judgement call. It is what medical professionals are paid to do, and what we are trained to evaluate and make a judgement call when assessing facts and data. But like the terms no and yes, no means no, and yes means yes. As the answer is either yes, a drug causes a complication, or no it does not cause a complication. "So what" is a yes, a drug causes problems and complications but may vary in the level of discussion among medical professionals who may feel only a limited need for having such a discussion. The "so what" crowd may easily slide to no as the answer given to patients, as concerns are considered not "serious enough to address" except in certain intellectual circles. Or perhaps, "so what" can easily be changed to a no for the right compensation. Doctors will often state "so what" in conversations with other medical professionals but will slide the answer to a no when acting as the well-paid government's expert in a courtroom. Is this news shocking to citizens? Citizens should be astonished; the voice of our government can restate a yes is really a no when it comes to an expert's statement regarding a vaccine injury. Why? Because they say so, and no further discussion of vaccine facts and science is allowed on the matter.

I suggest these are vital questions we as citizens must ask for clarification about vaccines, because the issues of harm are in some manner acceptable to many parties. Even as a "so what" statement should be addressed when the harm could have been avoided if the medical professional had just taken the time to learn the risks and how to address them. I stated this argument to our government, and the voices of our government say, "so what". Our government says a doctor knows what they know and can freely change their mind at any time. "So what" could be made off-the-cuff to other medical professionals and explained that yes he believed vaccine-triggered injuries happen and were important, but his concerns were not as important to him relative to other concerns and he could manage medical complications even though he had never addressed the complication at any point in his long career. A common highly overconfident statement made by many doctors. Then, without supporting evidence, later in time changing his answer to no, there is positively no evidence of the adverse event being vaccine-related, which was his last and final answer. What science would suddenly change an expert's answer, from yes to no? Nobody knows, and no science was presented to support the change in his answer. The question just resulted in disgraced silence, then a string of certain lies and super-defensive statements which it turns out were more lies anyone could validate as perjury. Anyone that is except for a special master it was learned. The "so what" argument is and always will be our government's position regarding many vaccine-related injuries, which has been a fact for two centuries, and addressing such vaccine safety issues are not on our government's list of top priorities.

I agree a professional judgement decision must often be made, but the argument cannot slide from yes to no. Unless the science suddenly shows the facts were in fact incorrect and proven incorrect through science. But in government arguments about vaccines, answers can slide from yes to no and back to yes in a moment without a discussion of facts. Some medical professionals and authorities simply refusing to address the changes in their expert opinion. I suggest all facts are worth discussing, and a child's risk of being harmed make it critical to discuss; and the parents are always the decision-makers, not the medical professionals and authorities trying to take that opportunity away from the parents using false and flawed arguments, which is unfortunately often the case with vaccines.

The parent is the voice of the child as children do not get to vote in deciding which medical treatment options are best. Medical experts do not get a vote and neither do government authorities unless the parents are absent or if the parents neglect their duty and hand the choice over to the government to decide. Today with vaccines, we are often told to be silent and let the experts give us the answers. The old-school methods of careful assessment and strategic planning are unfortunately not how our government wants us to act as citizens or as medical professionals.

The "so what" statement should be a major concern for all citizens. As all drugs have concerns for adverse drug reactions, and one class of drugs should not be excluded from following established drug safety requirements established in our nation's drug laws. And where such exclusion exist, should there not be a higher enforced standard for citizens to have access to information to make the important decisions on what the adverse risks are before administering the drug and the freedom to make what has always been known as a patient's, or parent's, informed consent decision. I do not hate the vaccine drug class. I simply demand higher standards for vaccines, as a balance to professional and government indifference. I find the "so what" statement highly insulting to me professionally and to all citizens who are in some fashion considered not smart enough to make an informed consent decision.

I, like many citizens, have not always had such concerns about vaccines. Trusting first my professional medically-trained parents would generally make the right decisions and believing that the doctors would always do their best to address all medical concerns which always filtered through my parents regarding my needs as a child. I was raised around medical professionals, and I learned to ask a lot of questions, and to in some manner trust the complete list of facts would be available. But as I have walked through the vaccine disaster program known as the VICP, I have found a better understanding of why a conflict exists for many citizens relating to vaccines. Why anti-vaxxers exist, and why many citizens reject vaccines for themselves and their children. Many vaccines are not the practical drugs they once were, as other drug therapies have been and continue to be developed as alternative drug treatment plans. Pharmaceutical research is full of great pharmaceutical discoveries waiting to be applied in medical treatment plans, but such scientific discoveries always have risks and are always addressed with better reporting literature to resolve any misunderstood risks and harm that can be caused to a patient.

What reasons do we, as a society, have for aggressively granting liability protection to drug manufacturers at the potential risk of causing harm to a child? For me there is no justification, if the risk is known and explained through scientific discovery and labelled as a drug ADR by multiple scientists. I do not need discretionary professional medical judgements by a government authority, or an expert acting as the voice of our government, to tell me I am wrong. "So what" is not an answer to the drug safety question. but is a question that must be answered by the person making the statement. "So what" can be an opening statement, as medical professionals understand the problems and ended with, we must seek the answers to solve these concerns. And not "so what" we should just disregard one set of medical complications, as one medical concern is more important than the other in harm caused to a child. One issue is primary and the other is secondary, and we cannot just disregard the secondary serious complications, because a medical professional determines the primary benefit far more important, or the primary risks as being only marginally important. For the record, serious secondary medical complications often cause more problems than the simple onset of a primary adverse vaccine reactions. In this "so what" mindset, secondary adverse events will never be adequately addressed.

It is true, vaccines prime the body to make protective antibodies. It is also true it will help the body form a protective immunity against a particular "foreign" agent, which vaccine antigens are designed to mimic. Everyone would love protective immunity to all diseases, but what are the individual's costs for such a comprehensive protective immunity? What are the tradeoffs? Does "so what" answer the concerns of a patient who is immunized will by design to develop protective immunity after several weeks hopefully against the right infectious pathogen, at the right time before the patient becomes sick from the pathogen, and hopefully it does not cause any serious adverse vaccine-related injury. Maybe just the small set of adverse complications such as the general feeling of being ill; and what about if the vaccinated patient develops serious complications? Vaccine experts understand vaccines are not 100% safe and mechanisms of action and mechanisms of injury are not fully understood, as some of the same mechanisms that trigger an infection can also trigger an adverse vaccine reaction.

The general concept involves immune system responses which trigger other body system responses. The same concept applies to all drugs. For example, just because you take a drug for a headache, does not mean it is not also hitting every other targeted pain or inflammation cell response throughout the body. Vaccines have a target, and it is often immune-system mediated cell responses, but vaccines also hit other cell targets like regulatory responses in the liver and spleen, and secondary responses like inflammation throughout the body. Vaccines are drugs, and patients do not get free passes to adverse events from any drug, without pharmaceutical intervention or favorable body responses. All drugs and all vaccines cause adverse events. The hope is the body after an adverse event will find a way to correct itself and return to normal function, but sometimes that does not happen, even as doctors try to intervene.

What are the immediate concerns in this scenario? Is "so what" the answer doctors often suggest as just hitting the reset button with some other drugs and the complications will get better or the body will figure it out if we keep the body systems stabilized. The answer the government offers through its experts, acting as the voice of our government, is exactly that, "so what" a major complication may happen from a vaccine, but the benefits of the vaccine are far more important to the expert, and by extension as the voice of our government, to our government. An injured party should not blame the drug for the drug is labelled as being safe and the doctors can fix the problem, because doctors are like God and can fix everything. This is where the "God-complex" statements begin, but do citizens really believe such statements of doctors can fix anything. If you are uncertain what the answer is, the answer is no, doctors cannot fix everything. In fact, sometimes they cannot even fix the simple things, as it is not in their realm of knowledge. We leave it to stupid lawyers to decide if it is within a medical standard of practice, as to whether to let citizens be permitted to sit and let a jury decide whether a doctor is liable for their notable ignorance. Or should vaccines have a "most favored" drug status among citizens who have come to accept the misunderstood adverse vaccine risks and bow to our government. The voices of government states "so what", if an adverse medical event occurs, that the adverse event is just unfortunate and if we lose the patient then that too is unfortunate.

This is the current voice of many of our medical professionals and the louder voice of our government. What is stated as a sound bite to end brief discussions, "so what" offers fewer efforts to seek answers to serious adverse vaccine-related complications and to learn lessons from other scientists and medical professionals in how to properly address the potentially serious medical complications. The ideas of science are thrown out, but demand on-the-fly judgment calls where medical professionals are left to deal with the more dire consequences later. Does this sound like science to you? Or does it sound like experts and a government that just wants you to do what they tell you to do. What they decide is the best thing to do. I detest the "so what" statement, and if I ever hear it, or other comments, like "whatever", or "well we just don't know what happened, or it is idiopathic, and we will keep an eye on it". Keep an eye on what? Our government claims both ignorance and superior knowledge at the same time. How are they going to keep an eye on a problem which has already been resolved? This is where I begin to ask a lot of question, because if the person stating "so what" does not know the answers, maybe someone else does, or at least the answers to the medical complication are discoveries waiting to be discovered.

At some point, scientists shift gears and become more focused scientists, and their scientific impulses kick-in. The scientific methodology requirements kick in: Develop a question that needs to be answered, research or find research of others that have encountered the same observed event, hypothesize what could be the answer to what is going on from experience and learned science. Experiment or see if other scientists have experimented and been peer reviewed as having reasonable and logical conclusions. Record observations and do they match observations noted. And draw conclusions, and do they match conclusions made by other scientists looking at the same problem. And finally, communicate and share results, and replicate if possible. The basic steps of research and science, which I have followed repeatedly.

I understand the "so what" argument and I believe most citizens understand the "so what" statement, but I have trouble with our government misunderstanding the statement and accepting an obvious yes a vaccine can cause a serious adverse reaction but "so what" a government expert acting as the voice of our government is not too concerned because the vaccine protection offered is more important than the adverse vaccine events, which a special master can simply overlook and state that vaccines do not cause these adverse vaccine events, but even if they do "so what". I really did not intend on having to address this argument in the VICP court, and I certainly believed I had the superior expert in Dr. Bellanti to explain the scientific medical facts. The question of this argument was raised as it relates to what the professional standards and drug actions are established through years of science and prior statements of expert knowledge, and what facts changed that common statement of concern among many experts.

My experts stuck to my son's adverse vaccine response and subsequent medical complications and treatment plans, which can occur and can become serious complications, and must be addressed to the best of a doctor's ability as an argument that yes, influenza vaccines can trigger nephrotic syndrome relapses and yes the medical complications can become serious and should be addressed as being related to a vaccine-triggered injury. The government's selected expert, a retired pediatric nephrologist Dr. Bernard S. Kaplan, started the conversation as an expert statement about medical complications, then suggesting a "so what" argument for vaccine-related injuries. I will post his video online for readers to watch, as the video is a legal document and was made in a public forum. Dr. Kaplan made the "so what" statement and argument at a NephCure medical conference in 2010. Dr. Kaplan had concerns about nephrotic relapses triggered by vaccines but stated "so what". Well "so what" became who cares and it does not happen, when Dr. Kaplan drifted to retirement and accepted his position to serve as a voice for our government in the VICP. In 2013, he stated with certainty vaccines do not trigger nephrotic relapses in an expert letter sent to the court in 2013, and he repeated his professional views in another VICP nephrotic case in 2016. A clear change in professional position in a short-window of time, from yes the medical complications are a concern to no, not only are they not a concern, but they have never been a concern.

Our legal question to Dr. Kaplan was, as it is with anyone that makes such a statement, is, what is "so what", and why did he flip-flop his expert medical statements of concern on several occasions over several decades. What and where is the science to support his newfound expert claims? What are the experts saying today, is it "so what"; or is it there is absolutely no concern for vaccine-induced relapses; or is it yes as explained in recent studies and even in medical office posters stating his stated original 1999 to 2010 concerns were in fact valid concerns related to vaccines? Dr. Kaplan did not answer the question in the VICP court, in fact he just lied, and lied, and speculated, insulting our expert who was not present, then lied some more. And asked to walk through a case report, which he said there were none that existed "anywhere in the world", but there are many noted case reports and clinical studies and not just one.

We demanded a discussion of science, and what were we missing, or better yet what had he missed. Despite our search for understanding and science that did not seemingly support his recent VICP claims to expertise, Ms. Millman assertively stepped in and prevented the discussion from going any further. Dr. Kaplan did not need to explain himself to her. She had the authority to independently give him discretionary forgiveness, without ever answering our question. I think this nonsense is sufficient to show the voice of our government, and especially the voice of the VICP, stands behind the "so what" claim to vaccine-related injuries. The government's experts, lawyers, agency heads, judges and special masters (the ones the Vaccine Act stated would be fair) all back the "so what" argument with regards to do vaccines cause many injuries, such as a nephrotic relapse which can become far more difficult to manage and complicated by a required change in treatment protocols, but who cares? Certainly not our government.

The science and the "expert" discussion in the VICP court did not supply any government science-based answers to these notable and sound vaccine-related injury concerns. I will share the details from the trial hearing and the transcript to the hearing online. Citizens can be the judge. Is our government a "so what" kind of authority relating to vaccine injuries, or is our government simply trying to hide the facts until at some point in future when facts become overwhelming. The question should be, is there a red line defined for vaccine-induced adverse events? The VICP and our government's red line is clearly ambiguous. The red line in medicine and science is much more defined. The National Academy of Science states a line that if a medical complication happens once somewhere, it is likely that it has happened many other times around the world. The answer is, we should address the adverse concerns now, not later, but now.

For your reference, Dr. Bernard Kaplan was not a novice expert, in fact you can detect his shrewdness in-person (again, I have the video). I imagine decades of being called an expert leads a professional to become confused and perhaps gives mixed statements. An expert should have the opportunity to correct themselves, but in the VICP there would be no required correction, just an arrogant expert going before the court and having an accident in their pants, and walking off the stand, which was somewhat satisfying, but did not answer any questions about the science or why he made these statements in the timeframe he made them, rather than a different timeframe he could not fully correctly recall. I would say in a normal court, a jury would have caught on to the lies and bias in the courtroom, and an unbiased jury would have rendered the right decision, in perhaps an hour or a day. But under the government's vaccine court special master system of discretionary decisions, discretionary actions are clearly screwed up and scientific arguments do not need to be fair. Ms. Millman did not take days to make a decision but took over 8 months to twist her facts. the maximum time allowed by court rules to form an insanely stupid opinion of the hearing and the science. And a clear fulfilment of her pretrial threat, and the opposite of her previously stated understanding of facts, in fact establishing new conclusions of science in the process of deciding a vaccine injury case.

It took Ms. Millman months to produce what must be one of the screwiest decisions ever in the vaccine program. A decision she obviously took her time in fulfilling her threat that we accept her random-offer sum settlement, that nobody knew the exact settlement amount, as it was an unreasonable settlement threat. Ms. Millman would go on to mislabel medical records, misstate and made errors on medical facts and medical literature including the case report we had hoped to discuss (which was added to the post-trial briefs as permitted), misunderstanding the causational mechanisms, and a long list of misunderstood facts and science. These records will also be available for readers to review and judge for themselves online. The saddest part is the child who was injured sat through the entire hearing and was ignored throughout these insane arguments and discretionary facts, and harmed further with stupid and insulting statements, which our Courts and government does not care to address, under their broad discretionary authority.

My son's case demonstrate the government and the voice of our government now takes the "so what" argument to the next level through the VICP court elevating "so what" to "who cares", as vaccine adverse events may happen but our government can reject them as if no one should care. A dramatic shift in the government's promised peace-making Vaccine Act legislative idea, and a biased shift to using paid government experts as shields to protect the VICP and vaccine manufacturers. I was fully prepared to give facts and engage in an aggressive discussion of science and facts, but clearly my attorney preferred the dramatic-staged methods of lawyering and simply staged a little baby-dance, like he accomplished something by playing a video and did not need to explain science or facts to his former special master fling. I simply had to scream, where the hell is my discussion on science, and facts related to my son's case. The government and our Courts simply state, "it is our special master's discretion to exclude these facts, and your son he can simply apply for welfare, and his family can address his future care needs".

Great job government, and great job lawyers, and great job government experts, the voices for our government. Not only did the government screw up a child's life, but they also changed science, and disregarded multiple principles of law regarding evidence and facts, in the name of protecting vaccines. What a shame our government has fallen to this new lowered level of authoritative discretionary actions to protect a drug class that is mostly unnecessary for most citizens. The "so what" argument has simply rolled into an argument of who cares, it happens, that is unfortunate, and what do we do now, accept all nephrotic injuries as being triggered by vaccines? Well, yes, admitting their errors would be a smart place to start, but that does not happen, and it did not happen as a matter of discretion all the way up to the Supreme Court, as I tested to see just how far this vaccine legal foolishness would go. Citizens should be genuinely concerned for their children and loved ones when science and false and perjured statements are made acceptable as points of law and science, and not actual discussions of the facts understood and discovered in science.

My son's case was the suggested outcome the special master had threatened prior to the trial hearing, and science was intentionally not addressed as the special master intended to find a path to her predetermined conclusion, which is also called being arbitrary and capricious. I hear government officials running around today saying, "we must follow the science", "the science is what matters" and "science gives us the answers", but they may as well be speaking from their other orifices because the voice of our government was loud and clear in the VICP and the Supreme Court decision to decline hearing facts and real perjured vaccine discussions. Science does not matter and harm to a child does not matter. For our government, the only thing that matters is vaccines and that vaccine manufacturers are protected from liability, which as a medical professional makes me feel ill, for my son and for all citizens. If citizens are concerned and want to help, spread the word, our government does not practice vaccine drug regulation and review of vaccine safety measures for the benefit of its citizens.

Ms. Millman retired after my son's case and left her final statement as a voice for our government on her way out the door, but do not assume things will get better as the program and authorities running the VICP are wildly inconsistent and wrong. If the VICP is drifting to being a welfare replacement program for disabled children and citizens injured by vaccines, the government should just say so and make it part of the stated law, so all the citizens can understand what the Vaccine Act really offers as a resolution to vaccine injury liability concerns. Or perhaps the government simply wants to hold off vaccine injury claims until the government's experts can catch up with the science, suggesting citizens are not too smart and it will take a while to figure out what is going on, much like they do with other laws, and how they eventually "worked out" the GBS concern from 1976 in 2018. Mix-up the message, change the narrative, and make the concerns political. Again, citizens must simply state "give us the science" and give us ALL the science. We cannot allow government authorities to manipulate citizens by abusing their power to shape the vaccine law into something they want and not something nature says must be understood through science. Citizens and parents cannot be restricted from discussing facts and evidence when our government supports false statements and misunderstood facts.

I argue we must fulfil our duties as citizens and certainly as medical professionals, and demand all parties come to the science discussion table and answer why scientists should feel the need to discard a discussion of science as a protection of their professional reputation to protect any drug and harm caused to children. Are vaccines exceptional and exclusive? My professional statement is, no vaccines are not exceptional, and any drug-related injury to any patient is an injury that must be addressed by our government. Ms. Millman and the VICP program did not hold a hearing six years after the injury claim was filed to settle a vaccine injury claim, but to endorse the vaccines with understanding of arguments that were false and harmful to all citizens. The VICP fills the void for addressing safety and injury concerns by filling a legislated gap with doctors that say "so what", vaccine injuries are not an important concern, and citizens do not need be alerted to the science.

Should citizens simply trust selected experts and our government because they suggest they know more than citizens that have concerns about vaccines and vaccine injuries. Our government suggests vaccine laws are of no concern to citizens until we have more solid evidence which they fail to provide. Delaying addressing adverse reactions until the medical community in this country, not other countries where the fact standards are already accepted, demands a change in addressing vaccine-induced injury causational mechanisms. For nephrotic patients that day may come. Dr. Kaplan and special master Millman gave us the accepted mechanism for causation of nephrotic syndrome following a vaccine, and the appellate and Supreme Courts affirmed the causational mechanisms through discretionary actions and confirmational statements. Future cases looking for a causational mechanism in the VICP should look no further for broader vaccine-injury nephrotic causational mechanisms. The cause of a vaccine-induced nephrotic syndrome state following a vaccine is now labelled as being caused by podocytopathy and has been accepted by the federal Courts as being caused by Angiopoietin-like 4 protein regulating factors. Do not mix-up the arguments, for the special master will surely mix them up for you. I will explain the details on this argument more online.

Our government has failed for decades now to address the concerns of individuals relating to vaccine safety and injuries using unfair and unjust arguments relating to using poor scientific methodology. Allowing lawyers and politicians to decide what the injured individual's fate should be, and not juries made up of fellow citizens. Allowing legal professionals with minimal scientific understanding of causes for vaccine-induced injuries to not only help craft the law, but also to administer, and play a role in dictating how the law is randomly applied to injured patients. What sounds like a great idea to many parties, sounds like a raw deal for an average citizen. Again, should we trust our government when they put their trust in experts like Dr. Bernard Kaplan and other VICP experts who state "so what" arguments and lacking enough confidence in understanding the science to actually dive into the discussion rather than take offense to his obvious lack of expertise.

As this was the government's approach and methods of attacking our experts and me. Petitioners are not attacked with facts but presented nonsense that had been addressed and accepted by the special master and DOJ since 2012, five years earlier, as understood facts. Why reshape facts for trial that had already been accepted five years earlier? Ms. Millman had no trouble changing facts or changing science to fit her decision, creating yet another isolated vaccine injury FIASCO which she has often brought to the table in her long career as a government legal professional. Other government authorities simply dismiss such arbitrary and impulsive actions as discretionary and unimportant to citizens.

And again, I do not want to leave out Dr. Arnold I. Levinson, Dr. Kaplan's UPenn colleague and long-time vaccine advocate and former member of the VICP medical board. Who was also exceptionally biased, and made many false statements in his attempt to clean up Dr. Kaplan's mess? Throw in a small group of DOJ attorneys addressing my son's case and you have over 15+ highly biased government voices acting as aggressive advocates for vaccines. Against my solo inept attorney was Mr. John F. McHugh, who for the record I honestly tried to find another VICP bar member attorney many times to take over and address the science. Our expert, Dr. Bellanti, understood the science, the medical condition and immunology perfectly well, in fact he wrote many of the textbooks on the science. Dr. Albert Quan, our other expert, could only make a brief appearance, as the court did not feel his presence was needed for more than a day.

By my count, the petitioner making a claim for a vaccine injury are considerably outnumbered in supportive experts and staff working for our government by at least a five to one (or more) ratio, and the government's voices are not independent or fair-minded parties but are aggressive advocates for vaccines. The Vaccine Act suggests the VICP special judges will function as a sufficient and unbiased finder of facts for individuals injured by vaccines. I firmly attest the VICP special masters offer little concern for injuries but slowly and methodically attempt to see if injured parties will accept a low-end settlement and give the vaccines a continued protected status by releasing the vaccine from any liability as the originating source of a vaccine injury. I have never accepted any such release of liability and will continue to fight to correct these errors and actions of our government. My facts and my son's facts relating to the vaccine triggered injury and complications are correct.

I give emphasis and point to many societies that have failed when citizens stop caring about individuals, and not just any individual but our children who are not full citizens yet. Children who rely on the parents and the government to teach and educate them as to what is right and what is wrong. Is the "so what" argument acceptable and is this what citizens consider the right message to teach our children. That is the lesson our government has instructed many citizens and told parents of disabled children in the VICP court to follow or else. Not let us look at the science and get it right but let legal authorities give the government's voices maximum clarity in its message to affirmatively promote vaccines. Our government takes science and forces it upon citizens as their only choice for public health and infectious diseases concerns. Even as vaccines are not the only drug options available to address infectious diseases. The government continues to work off promotional and protective actions the government considers necessary in some fashion to protect two centuries of being in a vaccine partnership with vaccine manufacturers. At some point our government must understand, No means No, and we do not have to take vaccines or else. Or else what? Take a better treatment protocol with better safety profiles.

Dr. Bernard Kaplan framed the need for vaccines perfectly but did not do so on purpose. His "so what" statement frames the government's message. Children will suffer harm because we need to "protect" them, even as it may also cause serious harm and injury. A child is young and strong, capable of bouncing back, and if they do not then that is simply unfortunate. An elderly citizen is old and frail, with a weakened immune system so our government must take actions which will protect these valuable citizens. Hey, I get it, I am getting older, every day; and "so what" is a move towards self-preservation and self-interest actions. But at what point do the citizens reject the government authorities' acts of self-interest and self-preservation and move forward with facts and arguments of science.

I was ready to argue science in 2016, and I am fully ready today. Let citizens demand facts and evidence that are transparent for all vaccines. Let us teach our children about vaccines and their place among all drugs and how they can cause harm to individuals, so they can teach their children the correct lessons. There is no need to hide the small scientific details, as the science will either explain the safety concerns or the science will explode. Or maybe the science already imploded in 1986, when the Vaccine Act was enacted using legal discretion and false promises for science as a basis for discovery. The "so what" argument has been shifted as relating to vaccines and the impact infectious disease have on older citizens with lessened immune systems, where protecting our elderly replaces the need among self-interested government authorities who rate their personal concerns as being more significant than the needs and concerns for our children.

If you are interested in the facts, video, testimony, and evidence from my son's vaccine injury claim and trial it will be available on my website, www.VNTY.Health (yes .health is a valid web link) . I can hopefully help citizens who struggle with many vaccine facts and Vaccine Inc fun facts and our government's approach to safety. There should be no arguments that vaccines can cause harm to any citizen and must consider a child who is growing and learning to become a citizen, noted as being a citizen-in-training. The "so what" argument to vaccine-related injuries is not a healthy alternative for public health or scientific discovery. I hope citizens check out the facts, as our government will not be offering the details to the public anytime soon. They would rather brush the dirt under the rug and move on, hoping everyone will read nonsensical judicial legal opinions as the government's fact statements, and ignore the actual case records and trials. I will never accept their garbage science or their garbage law, as the only answer to vaccine safety is equality for all citizens and equality for all science discovered and understood. And that all science about all drugs should be available and open to discussion to all citizens. A single child harmed and not properly addressed is one child too many, and the "so what" statements of our government, regardless of the source acting as the voice for our government, are never acceptable replacement statements for dismissing vaccine injuries.

CHAPTER 7

The Rights and Duties of Parents and Our Government

Once a citizen reconciles the "so what" argument and maybe you have that ridiculous argument settled in your mind. The next argument must be what are your duties and your rights as a parent, and did you know your government has an equal right and duty to serve and protect your child.

As an adult, at the age of 18, all citizens have a right to make health choices as they see fit; but up until that age, parents have a duty to guide in the protective development of an informed and capable citizen-in-waiting which all citizens hope will grow to be an informed and capable adult. The government has an equally important responsibility to make sure a child and parent have access to resources and are given the opportunity to assist the child in becoming informed adults capable of making well-informed choices. A parent can lose their rights to make decisions for a child, if their actions are judged to be harmful, incompetent, or negligent. A child does not have the rights and protections of the Constitution or many laws until they are adults and citizens, at least not citizen rights. Which party holds the most control over a child? Neither, as it is an equal duty to be a parent of a child and to be a government with oversight serving its citizens-in-waiting.

Adults and incapacitated citizens for assorted reasons may lose their rights, but in general after the age of 18, a citizen is expected to make informed and knowledgeable consent decisions. It is your choice to give up your individual right, to a government, or to a medical professional, to a neighbor, an acquaintance, or even a public health official. Some of these informed consent decisions are granted to others as laws of society or military service, but if an individual genuinely wants to make an informed decision that others may consider good or bad, it is the individual's right to make an informed medical choice. Such informed decision choices are the foundation of our government, formed under libertarian (not liberal) principles. The freedom granted under law to make informed and knowledgeable decisions. Adult citizens can make these well-informed determinations. Our government often strives to take away this right and freedom by suggesting they must intervene to safeguard all citizens.

Parents share the dual responsibility of making choices for their child, and while the government can mandate certain actions, the government cannot mandate actions which may cause harm to the child or harm to the parent. Other countries' governments may share an alliance with our government, but they too have no right or authority to direct any action or any decision-making for our citizens. This principle covers virtually all decision-making choices, as it is our law.

In a nutshell, this is your constitutional rights as an American citizen. If the parent neglects to perform their parental duties, the government can step in and make sure proper decisions and care choices are made for the child. All medical procedures and drug choices are in fact informed consent decisions to be made by the parent. No, not the "I don't know what this drug is" decision, or my doctor told me "to take this drug" decision, or my government recommends, or worse mandates, you take this drug decision. It is always an informed consent decision. It is a principle all citizens must understand. Citizens control and can use their brainpower to make fully informed choices and can also grant another party permission to make medical choices for you.

The proverbial "I do not know, you decide" choice is often a common example of this type of decision-making process. It happens every day, and despite allowing someone else to decide, as an adult you have in fact made your own choice. If the decision is good, it was still your choice. And the same goes for if it turns out bad, again still your choice. But as parents, it is again a divided choice for the safety and development of the child. First between two parents and then in partnership with our government.

Why is this important? It is important because it is an inalienable right as a citizen of the nation whose Constitution gives you those rights. In the case of a child, no one expects the child to have informed decision-making capabilities to make an informed consent decision, which may not be true for every child, but the law does not give a child full medical rights until they are 18, but does grant limited rights for healthcare decisions at age 13. The ability to sue or take legal action does not occur until age 18.

Why do I mention these rights? Because many Americans are confused by their rights and duties. And what the rights and duties of their government are in relationship to the citizen's individual rights. Or perhaps this is just a confusing time, and political players are shifting your rights, or attempting to take away individual citizens' rights. Again, our government often acts to intervene in the name of protection for its citizens and public safety, where the government must demonstrate a risk is certain and the protective action is the only solution, and not a "we think this is a risk" and "we suggest this is the only option", so fall in line or else, and if anyone gets harmed or gets hurt as our citizen, our government will fix it. This is not a solution but a false promise. A promise our government simply cannot fulfill and will always lead to failures and harm to citizens. I do not need to tell you this, as lessons from history will tell you this is how things left to our government to make decisions for our citizens often ends up as harming citizens.

Our government makes promises to its citizens and places demands on its citizens all the time, but it is the responsibility of the individual to make informed and intelligent choices, for if many individuals make intelligent and informed decisions, our society will be prosperous. If individuals make dumb decisions, for themselves and their children, society will certainly breakdown. As discussed in the previous chapter, does a child understand that they may be injured, and our government grants itself discretion to make a "so what" argument to their disturbing injury. Did the parent or child make the informed choice? No. Did you, as a parent, make an informed choice? Maybe, but maybe not, if proper information was not given to citizens by our government to allow citizens to evaluate and make an informed decision. Did the government authorities make a poor drug choice for citizens? Absolutely yes, as our government collectively and selectively supplies false guidance and drug information to all parties, and enticingly promotes liability protection to all vaccine-related parties. A problem arises as citizens are not properly informed what discretion really means in the eyes of a single specialized judge, and this discretion can be both harmful to citizens and children, and harmful to science and medicine as that single judge can distort laws of science to fit their preferred discretionary interpretations of the laws of society. This is not a third-party independent legal action by a group of active participants deciding for individuals what must be the law and forget about the laws of science for the laws of science are irrelevant in their eyes. The Vaccine Act was a law created, enacted, and shaped as a method of controlling citizen from storming against a specific commercial interest, vaccine manufacturers, with specialized exclusions, protections, and drug laws, which are not specifically allocated for protection of the citizens or children.

Our government does not offer individual citizens an independent voice relating to vaccine safety and vaccine laws. Our government appoints a single special master as being the sole legal professional with discretion regarding vaccine injury liability and designates a single expert a Patriarch of his profession to act as the government's voice on medical science. Our government declared Dr. Kaplan a Patriarch of nephrology medicine. A sort of crowning of an expert as the government's voice of facts and logic, but his crown is worthless to others, as some would consider him a fool. These are the actions our government takes to superimpose choices on its citizens. The government would not want citizens to think our government hires and promoters fools to preach their message and science but they do, as Dr. Bernard Kaplan lied, speculated science and perjured himself repeatedly, and made false assessment of my son's medical records. Government authorities have that kind of power, to change facts and endorse drugs as they see fit, not as the FDA and drug manufacturer report and publish as facts. All individual citizens have an equal power to make decisions and must use that power or lose it, for it is within the individual's power to also make informed discretionary choices at times when their health and their child's health are in danger.

Since 1986, the Vaccine Act has grown from actions and concern for protecting vaccine manufacturers from legal liability and incorporates a poorly understood legislated law to protect a massive vaccine industry. The vaccine industry has grown from a small group of vaccine manufacturers, to 50+ global vaccine manufacturers today, with varying levels of vaccine expertise and manufacturing capacity. And the vaccines are not just for infectious diseases anymore, as we now have vaccines for therapeutic treatments such as cancer vaccines and other specialized disease treatment protocols, many which are currently in clinical trials. The researchers of these novel vaccines hope and expect to one day be mass marketed drugs someday, and the question arises will our government also give these novel vaccine manufacturers a free pass to injuries caused by some of these eventually mass marketed novel vaccines with limited and discretionary liability covered by our government under the Vaccine Act and the VICP. The discretionary approval to grant liability protection and coverage is a possibility under the law, but where do citizens stand on requiring safety and science facts before endorsing any novel and unproven vaccine.

Pharmaceutical manufacturing capabilities and research of vaccines have also changed considerably in the last 30 years, but Vaccine Laws continue to address vaccines as having the need to be considered an exclusive drug class. Vaccines do not fit easily into other drug classes. Vaccines are a different but does not necessarily fit the meaning of being an exceptional and/or exclusive drug class. Vaccines are simply unique, and offer a choice which can be protective, but can also be harmful and unsafe. The decision to choose which drug choice fits an individual's life and lifestyle must be decided by the individual, and in the case of children by the parents. Our government cannot show where any vaccine is completely dependable or offers absolute protection, but a vaccine may demonstrate effective protection to a single pathogen.

As humans we are confounded by diseases and infectious outbreaks. There is always lack of preparations by many authorities and many professions for the endless healthcare needs of the masses. There is always need for medical care for the sick. And there is always death and disability. Is any party guilty of causing this current enormous health crisis? We may never know with certainty where the current COVID crisis was started as an act of nature or a failure of many parties. It may be convenient to point to a country as the source of the outbreak, but that is often simply a suggestive answer. As noted, the Spanish Flu was first discovered in Kansas, not in Spain or not even in a person from Spain. Infectious disease outbreak facts and arguments are often changed to fit a particular narrative or political story line. We may never have a definitive answer to many questions that science cannot easily isolate and answer. Some answers are simply not worth the cost to pursue or do not demand being answered, but some science deserves to be addressed as answers are not difficult and have already been answered relating to many adverse vaccine reaction concerns.

I mention these facts, as our government has tried to create answers and outcomes they wish for, in a political promotional narrative. Suggesting, do this and the authorities can make this happen. Like everyone wear a mask, and the virus will go away. As this claim is for the most part false, as we do not know that wearing masks and protective gear will be of much benefit, and if history is of any indication, COVID will be back in cycles for years and years, if not centuries ahead of us. The goal must be to limit infections in each cycle, where masks can help, but even the best masks are not 100% preventive. And neither is isolation and quarantine, but these actions have historically shown to be somewhat effective in managing the spread. Again, COVID-19 is highly contagious. It can be spread on surfaces, and through air at certain distances, and through animals, which means a lot of sources for catching the infectious disease. A mask and protective gear may help slow the spread, as does isolation and quarantine, but in the end history has always shown infectious disease will run in cycles and will require vigilance by the citizenry to manage and address the spread. And with proper treatment, a natural protective immune system may supply immunity to future infection by the same infectious pathogens. As your body's innate and acquired natural immunity are generally better than a manmade injected antigen triggering a protective response. God and natural science will always impart better tools than man and man's creative sciences, despite the beliefs and opinions of many who think otherwise. In random cases, governments have been part of great experiments, but the best scientific discoveries have come from individuals discovering natural science, generally with little or no support by our government.

Nephrotic syndrome is often regarded as a manageable but uncurable medical condition. There are no suggested cures, and our government does not offer answers or cures. Informed medical professionals offer hopeful treatment protocols. Our government impedes cures and selectively endorses medicine and treatment plans as they see fit under select guidance of a few designated nephrology "experts". Our government acts on science with actions that are often capitalistic actions intended to benefit the government, who claim an interest for all people, but are generally serving the interest for only a few parties and individuals. Our government has extremely limited interest in addressing or curing nephrotic syndrome. My son was once labeled an uncurable case of nephrotic syndrome but is now fully cured. I mention nephrotic syndrome for reference as our government offers suggestive scientific solutions yet rarely puts forth useful keys to a cure. They instead offer false hope. I simply say many individuals offer the answer to complex pathologically challenging problems, not our government. Our government is not a trustworthy healthcare partner for its citizens or for the science used in medicine that we search for as cures.

I do not believe we are at the end of humanity tied to an infectious disease outbreak as many citizens hastily claim. Is our current infectious disease crisis manageable, and do we have the resources to manage it? Again, I would say yes, we have the resources, but we should act diligently and intelligently to make sure all healthcare resources are used properly. Our government has repeatedly failed in supplying the necessary resources and services needed by many citizens to address healthcare needs. I can attest in the current crisis, as in past crises, our government has restricted and made limited resources available which are being underutilized and poorly organized and managed, which our government should be ashamed of for its inadequate management efforts. This is not a political statement, but a broad statement where all parties in government can share the blame and certainly the shame. Our government can simply take a knee to nature and stop throwing money at a force of nature we have little control over, but citizens can certainly band together and take actions that are lessons learned from history and lessons learned from science.

It is time now to slow down, review history, review lessons in science and other disciplines and to teach our children and our government (that often acts like children) how to get things done right. The duty of citizens, as it is with being a parent, is to educate and instruct our children. The duty of a child is to sit and learn and explore with only limited rights as citizens but a thirst for knowledge and discovery. The duty of our government is to manage and inform its citizens and to protect our legal rights.

Society and citizens should correct any individual or government who is incorrect in using discretion and false expertise as it relates to science, and correct a government made up of elected individuals who suggest an interest in representing its citizens but fails miserably at the task. Citizens protest and demand action when a harmful action against an individual or many individuals occur where an individual's rights are openly violated. Even as many citizens do not understand their rights and the rights of their children are often violated by many laws and actions by many authorities, including rights restricted by vaccine laws and programs. Correcting these harmful violations of rights do not demand a protest or violence, but simple actions that will enlighten our government authorities who oversees our individual rights and healthcare that we are in fact engaged and active citizens. We are citizens acting for our children and loved ones and in control of our constitutional rights which require we be informed and given facts for all drugs to evaluate and judge these facts for ourselves, and grant the same right to all fellow citizens to do the same in-depth analysis and evaluation necessary to make informed medical decisions in a fair and proficient manner. Democracy demands freedom must be granted to individuals to make well-informed and educated choices, and that all citizens be granted full access to all known and related drug facts.

CHAPTER 8

David vs. Goliath

Most citizens have heard the story of David versus Goliath. A biblical story of a confident individual named David who takes on a giant in the name of his people, and finds a way to win, because he must win, losing is not an option. I feel that way sometimes, but I am not going up against Goliath, I chose to stand-up to fight in opposition to a colossal Vaccine Inc, which is not a single giant but many giants that have grown enormous from government support and promotion. And the weapons used are not traditional weapons or political statements. The weapons needed to defeat Vaccine Inc are science. Who will check the science? Vaccine Inc and our government suggests they control the science, as they are our nation's legal validators of the science. Yet they also hide behind false scientific facts, which are obvious to any scientist that cares to look at the science and laws directed at regulating the scientific discoveries. Flawed laws and actions harm science and ultimately harms society as science falls behind and conflicts with scientists.

Most medical scientists understand the mechanisms of action of vaccines and understand vaccines can cause injuries and harm to patients, including the many scientists that are part of Vaccine Inc. Yet not all citizens understand the science and mechanisms of how vaccines work and can cause injuries as many citizens prefer to agree with the promoted idea that vaccines are generally safe drugs. Often not understanding vaccines cause many injuries and adverse drug reactions. Our Goliath feels no need to explain these mechanisms of injury, or that they even occur, and proudly proclaims, "I can do whatever I want, who will fight me". The answer is either fight our vaccine Goliath or shut up and accept the promoted directives the giant issues as laws. I, the little scientist, like David, with the slingshot full of science will fight our Goliath with vaccine facts and lessons scientists should have been addressing for our citizens all along. Goliath is big but Goliath can also be beaten, and citizens can watch or more successfully join in and show Goliath we are stronger together as a nation of citizens who believe in the mandatory need for drug facts and science.

Vaccine Inc is the current government bully on the block, and Vaccine Inc has a certain swagger. An odd swagger where they say they have us covered, and citizens should not listen to anyone else, and Vaccine Inc alone will protect us. Strange but this is the same message Vaccine Inc has been aggressively promoting since 1986, or 1813 if you want to return to the beginning of Vaccine Inc. For example, Alex Azar, the fifth Secretary of Health and Human Services in the current administration, states, "our agencies put vaccine safety at the highest level for all Americans". Interesting statement, but where were his army of vaccine safety teams during my son's VICP hearing or maybe he should have told the Courts "no, the Court's science is wrong", or "the special master is wrong, she has the science wrong, and she may be crazy". And why does FDA Commission Dr. Stephen M. Hahn, also the fifth of five FDA commissioners in the current administration, who currently pays no attention to the science adopted by the federal courts and turns a blind eye to a Citizen's Petition as mandated by law to be addressed in a judicious manner. The science adopted by Ms. Millman impacts hundreds of drugs with reported cases of causing nephrotic syndrome through what the FDA regularly lists as immune-mediated mechanisms, but the Courts now want to call it podocytopathy, misunderstanding the causation is actually called drug-induced podocytopathy, and in fact a lot of drugs trigger nephrotic episodes.

Podocytopathy is also a more current term used for nephrotic syndrome, and the term podocytopathy does not rule out immune-mediated causational mechanisms. Again, our government's chosen authority on vaccine injury decisions, Ms. Millman, got the science wrong, but she also changed the science for understood mechanisms of causation for nephrotic syndrome injuries. As the voice for Vaccine Inc, she did the science all by herself misunderstanding nephrotic syndrome science and adverse drug-related injury science, but government experts and special masters and judges can do that as Goliath gave them discretion to do whatever actions are needed to enforce the council (Congressional) laws. What's up Goliath, did no one send the memo out to all the heads of HHS agencies? And are their too many heads of too many agencies in the HHS empire? Or does Mr. Azar only read memos from select parties? It's okay Mr. Azar, we understand, you are we understand a businessman, not a scientist. Goliath only listens to internal business associates and politicians who can fire him or lead to greater treasures for himself.

Maybe Vaccine Inc's goal is to keep scientists off balance, and demands scientists follow the selected wisdom message being promoted by our government. Mr. Azar plays the current role of our authoritative stooge. He was the president of a major pharmaceutical company and on the board of a large biotech organization before becoming the Secretary of HHS. Do you think he does not have an interest in vaccines? Vaccines are in his past, present and future in some personal and financial fashion. In fact, many current government authorities are stooges, and those that cannot follow the political directives will be "fired" (put that on reality TV) or will often casually walk away to some cushy job somewhere else. The Presidential Cabinet that runs the enormous Health and Human Services umbrella of agencies has out-of-control discretionary powers which are now divergent from most citizen's interests.

The multiple voices of vaccine science in our government are not currently in harmony, in fact the agencies could use some teamwork to send out unified science, so the science does not become pointless and useless. For example, the VICP should listen to the FDA, since the FDA is our supreme drug agency; or is it the FDA should listen to the VICP as the Supreme Court states the VICP decision is a reasonable discretionary judgment that can use flawed science and biased expertise. Who is the authoritative expert in this maze full of false authorities under a single-umbrella Cabinet-member of the executive Presidential branch of our government? Is it Mr. Azar, a non-scientist, or Dr. Hahn, a seemingly excellent physician? Or are we counting on the cross-branch experts in the Judicial department to address science? The supreme authoritative powers in multiple branches of government are very confusing, and it is no wonder the scientific statements among authorities can get mixed-up. That happens a lot in a crisis, but it also seems to be an ongoing string of confused messages issued by Vaccine Inc since 1986, when the parties were supposed to join as one and help citizens that are harmed by vaccine injuries.

But instead all parties spend a lot of time nodding their heads in confusion and allowing each other discretion to further screw up the science. It is no wonder scientists, real scientists, have hesitated to address science in the U.S. with a lot of science being done overseas. For how can a scientist address science when authorities keep changing the scientific facts? Science and medicine are not the best business to be in right now, as regulations and discretionary oversight is harmful to both citizens and scientific professionals.

As noted, the Vaccine Act of 1986 gave nonscientific judges and special masters the power to dictate and rewrite science for the protection of vaccines, and not to address vaccine safety concerns for citizens. It must be understood the voices of our government, Dr. Kaplan and Ms. Millman, declared for legal argumentative purposes nephrotic syndrome is not caused by an immune-mediated mechanism, which was our VICP team's argument as stated in FDA literature and in nephrology textbooks. The mechanism is not exclusively immune-related, but clearly has immune system mechanisms involved, as the nephrotic condition is managed with drugs that suppress the immune responses in all body cell tissue. Dr. Levinson, the other government expert and voice for our government, agreed with the government's arguments by mashing up the science and drug actions of vaccines and other drugs. Ms. Millman being the brilliant medical-junkie judge that she thought she was decided for the sake of proving our argument wrong in her opinion, that Dr. Kaplan knew more than us, declaring podocytopathy (a new fancy term for nephrotic syndrome) was now the accepted cause for nephrotic syndrome, and our search for a cause to vaccine causational triggers was settled. To shorten the argument, podocytopathy is now used as a narrower and more specific term as a replacement for the broad term immune-mediated causation.

Podocytopathy was a term our side introduced to the vaccine injury causational argument in 2013, but Ms. Millman somehow forgot it was originally part of our scientific argument. Podocytopathy was also an argument used in another 2016 VICP case and wrongly dismissed by another special master, so in our trial in 2017 we stuck to the broader terminology accepted by the FDA and general nephrology textbooks. But in 2018, Ms. Millman declared the causation of nephrotic syndrome as podocytopathy, using mislabeled factors (labelled in court as angiopoietin-4, but is actually Angiopoietin-Like 4 or ANGPTL-4 proteins) that assist in regulating cell homeostasis, also known as balance in the proper functioning of body cell systems. Vaccines can affect this balance and cause a drug-induced podocytopathy (or nephrotic state if you are not confused by the two terms).

The experts in nephrology are not confused by the two terms, and I am not confused, but apparently the Courts are very confused, or they simply give wide discretion for special masters to misunderstand the causational mechanisms that cause drug-induced nephrotic syndrome caused by hundreds of drugs many which are still being researched and approved by the FDA. For example, the Pfizer cancer drug Sutent, yes the Pfizer making and distributing the game-changing COVID-19 vaccine, is used with cancer vaccines and notably causes nephrotic syndrome and other serious medical complications. Yet the FDA is fine with simply labeling the risk an immune-mediated complications and patients can simply stop taking the drug if doctors catch the complication. You know, the patient has cancer, and the doctors can figure out the nephrotic problem and fix it, or perhaps the patient was doomed to die anyway.

Pfizer's value as a novel vaccine researching manufacturer is now higher on the ladder of worth to our government, than any present worth of an individual's present value as a protected citizen. Under these value-based principles, our government allows authorities, like Ms. Millman to jump to flawed scientific conclusions and to misuse science. But who am I to tell the special master and federal Courts they are wrong? That job should fall to the FDA, the VICP's sister agency under the HHS, to inform the special masters the accurate facts on science about podocytopathy mechanisms, and someone needs to tell the Supreme Court Justices their lower court judges do not understand the science, or if they do understand the science, please explain it to the scientists who are still researching the mechanisms on the subject.

This is the type of nonsensical scientific arguments the VICP and Vaccine Act has created by assigning unqualified nonscientists to evaluate vaccine science, and relying on paid government experts who are often retired and not up-to-date in their scientific understanding, and perhaps should not be permitted to be the voice of our government and what they believe are discretional and mostly speculative matters, and are not openly addressed as serious scientific matters. I say, if you grab the banner and declare yourself the expert and the most knowledgeable person on the planet, regarding nephrology and science, you should explain the science to others, so all citizens will know how the science works, or at least properly explain the science if we are arguing scientific facts. Are these facts proprietary and secret so only a few scientists can know the facts? My facts are not secret, in fact you can find them online in the public domain. But our government believes no one must explain anything relating to our government's voices of expertise. Citizens should just shut up and be silent, which unfortunately is not in my scientific genetic temperament.

For the record, under Federal court discretionary actions, a special master, a Federal Review Judge and a panel of Federal Appellate judges have all declared, and the Supreme Court Justices agrees with the decisions through discretional disinterest in vaccine facts and science, that all forms of nephrotic syndrome are now understood to be caused by podocytopathy mechanisms related to ANGPTL-4. There should be no future misunderstanding in the VICP court and the government should apologize to the Rus family and their injured child, along with their nephrology expert (a German doctor) who explained podocytopathy mechanisms to the court's special master and Dr. Kaplan (who did not fully understand the science in 2016), misunderstood the causational mechanism of drug-induced nephrotic syndrome which retrospectively should have been accepted and ruled in their favor as a factor that causes vaccine-induced nephrotic syndrome.

Going forward, based on this newly VICP accepted causational mechanism, may all nephrotic cases in the VICP use these understood causational mechanism facts, thanks to the advanced scientific research and conclusions of our nonscientific friend, Ms. Millman and the Federal Circuit Judges Dyk, Moore and Taranto that contributed, along with the government-appointed voice of American nephrology and our government's nephrology expert as designated by our government, retired Dr. Bernard Kaplan. Can we all give them a hand for their fine scientific research and jumping in to show scientists at the FDA and other research facilities how it is done right in our government's justice system. Where the FDA and drug manufacturers are still stuck on the immune-mediated causational mechanisms for drug-induced nephrotic syndrome. I have been working on getting this causational mechanism corrected, so any patients that suffers a nephrotic or other ANGPTL4 (or other cell-to-cell mechanisms) related injury from a vaccine or other drug will now understand what the causational argument should be, which the FDA paradoxically seems to be having trouble addressing at the moment.

My FDA Citizen's Petition, arguing the science of the Court's accepted science, is stuck in neutral and is having trouble being addressed with all of this other important science going on to get a vaccine out the door at warp speed, but perhaps allowing approval of a COVID vaccine that is not safe and can likely cause vaccine injuries, which could be a problem if our government is not even addressing one of the noted vaccine injury concerns given to them by their in-house experts, right in their face. COVID-19 vaccines, like influenza vaccines, will likely trigger ANGPTL4 regulated vaccine-induced nephrotic syndrome onset and relapses in some patients, often in children who are most likely to have been labelled as having an idiopathic nephrotic condition. Hopefully, these vaccine injuries will now be properly addressed and vaccine injured patients can one day file a VICP claims to apply this newly understood VICP causational mechanism for a vaccine-related nephrotic injury, presumably applicable to all vaccine-related nephrotic injuries. It may take some time before podocytopathy and drug-induced nephrotic syndrome get accepted and listed on the Vaccine Injury Table, so be prepared for a long wait and argument on the science where the special masters can freely misunderstand and manipulate the arguments on science for their personal biased opinions until the science becomes more clear.

I state here I am not a translational research expert, but I can use translational pharmacy research to explain science, which is the professional skills used to build on basic scientific research to create new drug therapies, protocols, medical procedures, and diagnostics. I do not have the designation of being an authority like our government's authorities or any special ability to change science, but I can certainly read multiple studies, case reports and scientific explanations of drug reactions and relate them to everyday citizens. I make no effort to change or reinterpret expert researchers who have worked in the drug research field for years and generally give multiple references and peer reviews to back up their work. Citizens should demand our government do the same, at all government agency levels, and as required in our drug laws when evaluating drug safety, including vaccine safety.

So, if lawyers and authorities do not understand the science, can they make promises to enforce laws using any methods they like? That question is a question only citizens can answer. Discretional science does not lead to safe drugs or fair and just understanding of causational mechanisms in a Vaccine Injury courtroom or at the highest Court in our nation. The government's promise to address vaccine injuries are an empty shell of many flawed facts and flawed discretion. The core argument is almost an elementary school playground level argument, which I have pushed to the FDA to address, but the FDA is a bit busy and unable to address this science as it has a full plate regarding pushing out a vaccine at warp speed, which coincidentally could trigger several drug-induced adverse drug reactions, including drug-induced podocytopathy.

But do not fear, your fearless Justices of the Supreme Court are okay with discretional justice, even if it laced with lies, false evidence, and hints of large doses of vaccine-flavored bias. As you can imagine the science is complex, and I introduced the science to the special master but was not given a platform to discuss the science in a court of law. Ms. Millman stole that platform and used it for her own biased actions. Ms. Millman proved government authorities can be both wrong and granted discretion to decide whatever they want using their "logical" indiscretions to decide science based on their own beliefs and opinions. Ms. Millman it should be remembered did help establish what the VICP platform should be and how vaccine injuries should be compensated, citizens are simply small-minded minions in her government-controlled vaccine world.

So, citizens may ask, what does it matter if government authorities are wrong? Citizens are often not scientists, and many citizens do not want to see the science. Just tell citizens if a drug or vaccine is safe and whether it works. Citizens can get information from the medical professionals who are educated and paid to understand the science. The reason this problem matters is the science has been slanted in favor of vaccines for many decades now, and the science does not match what is understood by empirical observed evidence. As with other laws, if the scientists cannot explain the science, and operate on different assumptions and theories, because the science is not fully understood by all scientists, then the understood science does not move forward and does not get used to address many concerns, like vaccine safety concerns.

Vaccine Inc and our Justices do not care to address science-related problem, which elevates the risk level for citizens to develop such vaccine science-related injuries, and makes the science stagnant, as flawed understandings often perpetuates ignorance and false claims by the government, not answers and solutions. In other words, poor communication by multiple parties does not equal better science for citizens or the medical professionals giving advice to citizens, it is a slippery slope to bigger problems down the road.

If citizens want facts to match across many platforms and agencies, citizens must demand changes; but do not expect much in the way of changes, as big government rarely has the resources, the interest, or funds to make needed changes. And authorities do not have the political drive (generally a money thing) to make the changes happen. As vaccines received exclusivity in 1986, few parties stood in the way of the new law, but if the ball keeps rolling down the hill, many individuals will eventually be harmed, which is not a statement to create fear but a statement of fact and history.

Citizens must seek to understand the science, take note of therapeutic options, and safety and efficacy issues related to each infectious disease treatment option, and then make a discussion based on the value each option offers as a treatment plan. And if citizens want to leave it to experts, then start including experts in the field of expertise being discussed. Doctors are not experts on vaccines. Pharmacists are the experts on drugs. And drug manufacturers, including vaccine manufacturers, are experts but also must address all drug-related marketing reports related to their adverse risks in a timely fashion. The FDA currently does a poor job on addressing these concerns about all drugs, and an exceptionally poor job in addressing injuries and adverse drug reactions related to vaccines. Vaccine manufacturers rarely make any exceptional efforts to disclose newly discovered adverse injury concerns in the U.S. related to vaccines. Often suggesting they are "dedicated" to ensuring vaccine safety for patients, for which I simply say, "Right, the manufacturer's doctors are loyal to their Oath to put patients first, but fail in their practice to follow through on such promises". Again, look at the Pfizer drug example given earlier as a point of reference. You cannot argue both sides of the coin, one for safety and one for profit, are correct answers in a flip of the coin, which is what Vaccine Inc suggestively tries to do.

The mechanisms of action for vaccines are understood but are not fully addressed relating to vaccine safety. Suggesting, if scientists knew the mechanisms, they could fix it, but how can a scientist fix something they do not care to recognize as an issue. Vaccine safety concerns are that kind of problem, which makes vaccine-related injuries a long and costly risk evaluation process that is difficult to manage. Drug safety evaluations are a long and time-restricted assessment process for all drugs, so what makes the process different for vaccines? Vaccine's inner body adverse reactions are difficult to isolate yet are becoming more widely researched to isolate the causes of the adverse vaccine reactions. Some vaccine adverse reactions have in the past been overlooked as a discretion and ignored for decades, as not important enough to address. Why bother digging deeper, as there are no immediate legal liabilities to argue on the science, the Vaccine Act protects against these liabilities.

All drugs, such as antibiotics for example, are mandated to follow stricter drug laws and regulatory approval guidelines for safety. Vaccines are given special privileges as drugs, suggesting vaccines are "special" drugs and a lot of government money is poured into vaccine research and safety measures. Over the years, I have talked to some of these top vaccine scientists in multiple companies and agencies, and can state without a doubt, they have no clue how to address some vaccine injuries, or maybe they were just playing dumb regarding many vaccine injuries, including the injury I pursued as being a more obvious vaccine-related injury problem, nephrotic syndrome relapses, which has been caused by many drugs, including vaccines.

As noted, newer classification methodology for nephrotic syndrome has shifted a causational mechanism to list numerous drugs as triggers that cause what is known as drug-induced nephrotic syndrome in many reported adverse drug reaction cases. Sometimes these adverse reactions are listed as being uncertain as to which factor triggered the abnormal kidney response, but such responses are often thought to be related to a dosing or metabolism response which has not been fully addressed in research. Researchers will often point to the liver and drug elimination routes as in some fashion impacting multiple organs, which the kidney and spleen are often thought to be directly involved in the mechanisms of causation. And rather than attempting to address these concerns, the affected human subjects are usually removed from the clinical testing project and are told to avoid drugs in the same drug class, as it is too complex of a medical problem to address. There is no need for manufacturers to dig too deeply into the science but simply label these reactions as an idiopathic or atopic reaction, as they do not fully understand what is going on internally in the body systems, nor do they care to understand. Today some of these adverse drug reactions are becoming more sincerely researched by translational researchers, and the causes are tied to areas of body function which can be controlled and can be treated or prevented, but manufacturers and government authorities prefer to play foolish games and hold off on addressing the serious adverse concerns until the injuries grow larger.

The concerns related to vaccines are often pushed aside as adverse events that are not addressed under some hidden research process that citizens cannot easily access. I, for example, accessed a lot of vaccine data through clinical research data on novel vaccines which are more easily accessible, if you know where to look. Protective vaccine drug safety reporting is not held to the same open and transparent reporting methods as standard drugs, or even novel vaccines in clinical research stages. I have seen private research on vaccine research squashed for trying to address an adverse event occurring in protective vaccine patients. For what purpose? Because the government and manufacturers did not like the suggested science or causation being related to vaccines. But science today is pointing to more complications than previously accepted as being related to vaccines as being the causational mechanism for many adverse reactions which can then lead to additional more serious medical complications.

These are not the kind of regulatory and research discretionary actions one would hope for when looking for answers to problems in science, but increasingly such actions are more common when our government is involved in the process of offering suggestive answers to complex problems. We can call this dumbing down the science, which is not helpful or useful to anyone, except those that profit from a chosen set of suggestive facts and promotional science points-of-view. Hiding science does not open paths to answers.

These concerns are not specific concerns related to a single medical syndrome or condition but cross many organs and adverse complications which are found to be both short-term and long-term in how an injury can affect the body's function. If we permit our government to ignore or put a hold on science, citizens and medical professionals may never understand the science to fully explain adverse vaccine injury risks, as vaccine injury risks are currently protected from accountability. The research for drug effect discoveries is an endless circular investigation of a drug's action for beneficial actions that are wanted and adverse events that are undesirable, but at what point do authorities demand addressing reports of specific adverse events. These are critical and important questions that must be answered to fully understanding the vaccine drug science, as the lag time and the lack of aggressive actions in reporting by the FDA is well known to be a major concern to medical professionals.

Much as Goliath had his followers, because you know he was big and scary and demanded respect. Goliath's size and indifference can also be defeated, and science can defeat our Vaccine Inc Goliath as science will eventually catch up to vaccine injuries and will make the Vaccine Act obsolete as vaccines should be held to the same standards of safety and efficacy as all drugs. The question is not how but when will science and vaccine-injury science come together and show citizens our government has been lying to us for years and covering up their lies with false promises and false facts. And how many more citizens must be injured by vaccines that could have been prevented if properly addressed in science, or simply pursued as science rather than waiting for the science to hit the right authority in the head. Citizens can wait a few decades and scientists will work out many vaccine injuries someday. Would it not be ironic if Goliath had the adverse drug reaction, and no one cared to rush to judgement in addressing his medical concerns? Someone in the future will figure out the odd reaction of how he collapsed when he was hit square between the eyes with a shot of science.

The core weakness to our collective Vaccine Inc is the Vaccine Act. The Vaccine Act promises science and kindness but does not explicitly address the core science of vaccines. The law sets up a philosophical debate, not a science debate, which citizens can decide on addressing or perhaps ignoring, or simply leaving Goliath to decide what actions are best for citizens, and are vaccine injures valid or invalid relating to discretion and not science. The Vaccine Act crafted by Ms. Millman and fellow DOJ team members, and hammered out by politicians under pressure to find a legislative tool to fix the Vaccine Inc self-inflicted 1976 vaccine fiasco problem, and not by tweaking the broader FDA drug safety laws, our government reshaped our perspective of vaccine safety by permitting special legal interdictions.

Do citizens understand the many quirks in our drug laws? The layers and layers of drug laws crafted to give authorities discretion in how the laws are to be applied. If the citizens do not understand drug laws and laws created for public safety, how can citizens be expected to understand the Vaccine Act, and understand vaccines and other drugs are not on the same playing field but are playing by a different set of rules manipulated by using discretion, which are flawed applications of drug laws relating specifically to citizen safety. Our government authorities have granted vaccines their special permission as being essential and superior protective drugs, but our government does not require the same level of understanding of how adverse vaccine injuries can occur and the need for required research as other drug classes must address in pharmacovigilance post-approval marketing reports to the FDA.

Our government has decided for citizens that vaccines are vital to our societal existence. We cannot exist as a society without vaccines. A similar concept to water being a vital drug. Water is vital to all living creatures. Water is also a drug that is vital to the body's functional chemistry. An overdose of water (drowning) is bad, and too little water (dehydration) is also bad, but the therapeutic range of water use and the body's needs are broad. Medical professionals understand the relationship and usage of water in addressing the body's need for appropriate levels of water, and how it affects other organs and body function, but sometimes it is not as simple as adding or subtracting, but also knowing which reactions will occur and to provide supportive measures to keep the body in balance.

All drugs, including water, can cause adverse body system reactions and vaccines are no different from all other drugs. Our government however has demanded scientists treat vaccines as different under the exclusive protective umbrella of the Vaccine Act. I suggest here, if vaccines are vital or superior drugs when compared to other drug options, let the citizens decide which treatment plans are best and do not let the Vaccine Act stand in the way of making fair independent evaluations. The Vaccine Act was demanded by vaccine parties as a protection to vaccine manufacturers but is also a disservice to citizens related to vaccine drug safety and research to understand vaccine-related injuries.

If citizens demand vaccine safety, vaccines must be held to the same standards as other drugs. Does this mean the vaccine class of drugs will eventually go away as a protective drug choice? This is possible, as suggesting the cost to research and develop and to cover liabilities relating to injuries will spiral out of control. Vaccines must address safety and effectiveness openly and transparently and report drug data, to fairly evaluate their value as part of an infectious disease strategy utilizing all infectious disease treatment protocols, and related to all understood and suspected adverse drug reactions and harm caused to citizens.

All drugs have safety reporting requirements and standards for approval and regulatory follow-ups. The FDA has suggested they actively regulate vaccines, but I must state they do an extremely poor job of addressing vaccine safety, and applying normal drug safety standards to vaccines, where discussions are often held in a nonpublic forum not accessible to all citizens. A world without the Vaccine Act would simply mandate manufacturers follow the same rules for vaccines as are required for all other drugs. Would this result in fewer vaccines? Possibly yes, as fewer manufacturers would not want to pursue the risks of manufacturing a vaccine with higher cost due to vaccine-related injuries. Yet novel science has been used to advance vaccines as potential answers to infectious diseases and novel treatments, by suggesting a path for therapeutic uses of vaccines which are different from protective uses for vaccines. The excitement surrounding vaccines is no longer excitement for protective features of vaccines, except in an infectious outbreak, but what can be done with the discoveries made relating to the therapeutic discoveries, by pushing forward the benefits but minimalizing and marginalizing discovered adverse actions in therapeutic clinical trials. The Vaccine Act makes vaccine research a suggestive frontier for discovery but fails to address many adverse vaccine-induced injuries. For citizens who accept a drug that offers some very serious risks of injury as being acceptable for protection, must also understand the same risk of injuries apply to vaccines being developed for novel and commercial gain. Are vaccines a superior drug class relating to infectious disease management? Not really, as other drug research and need for drug development exists which is equally vital to future infectious disease treatment protocols.

Vaccines could not stand alone and survive as a drug class in 1986, but vaccines can survive without the Vaccine Act today and should be conditionally allowed as drugs, but must be mandated to follow the same drug safety guidelines as all other drugs must follow as a path to recognized benefits and also understood adverse accountability-covered risks. I suggest the legal tool used for control of our rights to choose a best option being used by our government is the Vaccine Act, as our government manages and controls

Vaccine Inc. There is a critical need to stop citizens from being controlled by our Vaccine Inc giant. If citizens want suggested protection by using a vaccine and accept all reported risks of possible vaccine-related injuries, let citizens have the freedom to make such informed choices. And if citizens want to be experimental lab animals for therapeutic vaccine research, again with understood risks, let them also make those choices. But under either scenario, it is appropriate that the Vaccine Act and the VICP and related vaccine programs should breathe their last breath of life and science can be freed to address all vaccine-discovered adverse reactions as scientists and citizens see fit, not as authorities see fit to allow and report under discretionary actions.

Our government has a policy they consider set in stone, and a protective Goliath apparatus they believe will protect their prized vaccines. Individuals, like David, however, have personal rights and morals, and the right to say no thank you to Vaccine Inc. Our government pours billions of dollars a year into vaccines, yet citizens receive a poor return on our investment. What better choice for addressing a flawed law than simply defunding the law, by simply walking away and leaving the government to address poorly made promises and funded actions they created. It is a citizen's right to make choices of drugs they chose for good health; but any citizen not at risk or citizens that have natural immunity do not need not be vaccinated, and can also address the concerns for infectious diseases utilizing other drug treatment strategies, including simple isolation and protective gear, and other drug classes with more researched and reported safety profiles, and always remembering that more drug information usually means better health outcomes.

Science and the consumer marketplace pick drug winners, but when science is ignored our government is picking the commercial winners. Today, the vaccine marketplace is segmentalized among regional and national interests, as some governments do not trust each other to address vaccine safety for their own citizens, or take actions that suggest they are playing a vaccine "arms" races to be first to find a suggestive discovery of a protective and safe vaccine which can be proclaimed a vital restorative cure for an implied risk to humanity. Citizens should not get caught up in games of politics and commercial games but must act in their individual interests as related to health and science that is discovered and reported in medicine, with full answers and data, not limited and restricted data. Citizens must demand safety and demand facts, and demand the facts be fully transparent and addressed or simply reject the vaccines which are not shown to be safe or clearly offering facts and evidence, and are not fully shown to be needed for fighting an infectious disease, which can be addressed through simpler and more transparent drug treatment plans. Citizens have options and hopefully individuals can help show citizens the path to answers to our health and drug problems, including defeating giants. Some giants must simply perish to move forward and make progress for both science and shared interests for all citizens.

CHAPTER 9

Individual Citizens vs. Authorities

Groups of citizens have often opposed laws and ideas advocated by leaders and authorities since the beginning of civilization. Entire nations and societies have fallen on miscalculations and poor decisions of authorities and leaders. The ideas of where strategic ideas come from in a democratic society and which ideas should be adopted in society ultimately falls to the individual citizens. Many political arguments lead to lost individual rights. To protect these rights, citizens must reject the authorities' actions and demand their rights to make informed choices.

As I previously suggested in history, citizens often look for authorities who prove greater knowledge and push-forward opinions suggested as being the best solutions to a concern. Nations are formed on the trust of citizens in their leaders to make confident and strategic decisions. This trust is written into laws and authoritative actions which grant some authoritative discretion, until citizens decide the discretion is too mixed-up and has been misapplied. At which point, individuals must act and demand transformation in the flawed laws and formally reject the authorities' poor ideas and discretions previously granted.

Citizen concerns are often based on both scientific and philosophic questions. The Socratic methods of debate were developed in early civilizations to debate ideas and address concerns using questioning and answering arguments to set up the best logical solutions based upon critically analyzed ideas. Authorities often tried to establish logic and knowledge based on good faith efforts to settle arguments. Unfortunately, the science and logic learned by such methods was often slow and authorities continued to make poor judgments.

Niccolò di Bernardo dei Machiavelli, a noted Western philosopher, proclaimed the need to approach leadership and political actions differently. Machiavelli suggested great nations are based on great ideas of strong leaders who act on ideas proven through groups of citizens called factions. Factionalism resulting in multiple sets of arguments and often arguments and solutions based on a natural set of laws using lessons learned in nature to develop knowledge. As an example, Rome had earlier used the confrontational methods of allowing factions of citizens and authorities to co-exist in unrest, suggesting better laws and understandings of nature and science would come from such natural disagreements and eventual resolutions.

But the balance of laws of nature and the interests of leaders and authorities often fail in times of crisis. Machiavelli stressed both the need for strong leaders and factions that generate ideas that supply checks and balances that lead to good governance. Machiavelli's ideas and philosophies set up the basis of many legal governing doctrines, including the United States Constitution. A strong nation is one that embraces the ideas of many factions or individual leaders.

In a free society, all citizens do not have to agree with the decisions of authorities or agree with actions based on self-interest and laws written by self-proclaimed experts who simply believe their beliefs and knowledge are superior to other individuals and factious groups. Authorities argue laws for society but do not also address citizen concerns and the laws of nature. In their actions and arrogance, authorities often shift from being authorities to becoming Noble Liars. Noble Liars acting as controlling authorities who freely lie to the citizens believing the citizens are not smart enough to make decisions and informed choices on their own. Rejecting Noble Liars is the basic idea that was first used in the formation of democracies and providing individuals basic freedoms. Citizens must be allowed to make proper and informed decisions when confronting different possible outcomes. To make progress and seek answers to the problems a society must consider.

I offer citizens proof our authorities today freely make uninformed decisions that harm our democracy and our nation's founding principles, and abuse many of the factions that make up of our nation. Many citizens do not understand the decisions and laws made by our Noble Liars. Factions of citizens with understanding of nature and science give way to philosophical factions that simply want to offer discretionary ideas and opinions, suggesting we do not need to understand the science because the Noble Liars can tell the citizens what works and what is best. This cycle of Noble Lies may work in short cycles, but eventually the cycle is broken by acts of nature which cannot be controlled by such absurd actions. As applying science to solve a solution is not simply applying one's opinions or beliefs but involves groups of scientists testing and using scientific methods to resolve misunderstood arguments.

In moments of uncertainty, some individuals will freely come up with answers, like trained medical professionals that are prepared with treatment plans and safe protocols before the crisis. Some individuals will be scientists that demand science that follows scientific methods and testing procedures that must be applied in seeking answers. Other individuals will simply look to fill the void of knowledge with discretion and assumptions based on what they think is the best choice. Noble Liars will look to squash individuals who are not in agreement with their solutions. Individuals must evaluate carefully what authorities say and what proof they offer as science. Ideas can be newly discovered and tested science, or ideas can be learned from science and historical events.

I again mention history and scientific methods as they relate to vaccines and the Vaccine Act. As the Vaccine Act is a relatively new law, which was formed not using scientific methods or history, but falsely suggesting vaccines had a safe and sound history and provided safe vital protection to all citizens. Vaccines had proven protective immunity could be developed through a normal immune process with the introduction of similar less threatening infectious materials the body would recognize as foreign. No equivalent scientific effort however had ever been made to fully discover and address adverse vaccine safety concerns. In fact, the Vaccine Act did not demand vaccine manufacturers address vaccine safety as required under standard Food and Drug laws citizens had accepted and adopted.

The Vaccine Act does not require vaccines to be safe drugs but continued the historical promotional practices of authorities to support vaccines as a favored infectious disease drug. The Vaccine Act did not demand medical professionals address the need for awareness of adverse vaccine reactions, but instead gave them incentives, liability protection, and support to help promote vaccine protection. The Vaccine Act fills a notable void that vaccine science and manufacturing cannot meet as required under conventional drug laws. Citizens and medical professionals were told the Vaccine Act was a solution that would fill the void and keep a "vital" drug available at the specific point in time, but made no attempt to address the groups of scientists that sought answers for vaccine-related injuries observed in everyday practice.

Citizens have long accepted vaccines being made without restrictions under a capitalist model system with absolute government support, which is an odd pairing. The characteristics of capitalism include capital accumulation, competitive markets, a price system, and the recognition of property rights. Vaccines under tight control of the government offer none of these characteristics but are held as being developed under capitalist and democratic values. There is little capital accumulation by private parties, a limited competitive market to demand safety and innovative ideas, a weak price system, and limited recognition of property and personal rights. The Vaccine Act itself is a flawed law to begin with, as misunderstood science is not quickly fixed as would be normal in an ordinary competitive market, and authorities restrict factions of citizens from freely pursuing discoveries and answers to the problems that made the law necessary to begin with, to give authorities discretion and Vaccine Inc parties a shield from liability.

The Vaccine Act does require individuals be supplied facts and evidence which will help them become well-informed citizens. The FDA uses discretionary science and deceptive good faith effort practices to help all Vaccine Inc parties push a vaccine promotional message that vaccines suggestively protect the citizens and are generally safe drugs, without ever diving all in on vaccine-related injury concerns. Good faith practices are short-term solutions but cause exponentially greater harm to individuals long-term.

Vaccine authorities have regularly bridged data and logic to fill voids in scientific data, as it has become obvious bridged data is required to approve new vaccines, to bridge the gaps in changing biological adverse reactions which cannot be determined in a short window of testing. Authorities have often opted to overlook vaccine injury concerns as a discretion, promising to address the concerns later. One of those "later" dates has arrived regarding GBS and its injury linked to influenza vaccines, which took a little over 40 years to address as a vaccine-related injury. Was the "later" GBS decision an acceptable and reasonable timeframe for evaluating and deciding a vaccine injury mechanism of causation? A recognized vaccine-related injury in 1976, but not a recognized Vaccine Table injury for decades. Citizens should figure out whether authorities took satisfactory steps to address a serious adverse vaccine reaction, where steps taken were slow and shifting and provided inadequate and restricted access to information and evidence to citizens.

Medical professionals must demand vaccine authorities acknowledge a citizen's right for access to all facts and information which is needed before informed consent is asked. Authorities push and promote the benefits of a protective vaccine but completely ignore vaccine safety concerns, suggesting an absolute need for the vaccine. Vaccines however do not guarantee eradication, which can take centuries to reduce and end a single threat of a viral pathogen. Smallpox is now thought to be eradicated, with the last reported case in 1980, approximately 20 years after an aggressive program to eradicate the infectious disease began in 1959, but over two centuries after Dr. Jenner's discovery. Smallpox viruses still exists in labs, and can still be a future threat, but is now easier to isolate. This eradication program forms the basis for most new vaccine programs authorities point to as a successful program and a success we must pursue for all infectious diseases.

Again, many infectious diseases are fully treatable with antibiotics or other therapeutic options. And smallpox did not fully undergo extensive testing about any adverse concerns. Pharmacovigilance and drug safety reporting studies were limited until the 1950s and did not became more focused until the 1980s. The Vaccine Act has walked back the required drug safety reporting standards for vaccine safety concerns and has created a barrier to properly address vaccine injury causational mechanisms.

The Vaccine Act has allowed authorities to openly claim vaccines are safe drugs, even as scientists are observing and demonstrating mechanisms of causation for vaccine injuries. The Vaccine Act has become not a law for the citizens, but a law to restrict individuals from understanding the actions of authorities. Authorities use naïve citizen indifference as a tool to press authoritative discretion to its limits.

Greater authoritative discretion does not equal better healthcare for all citizens. Authority cannot make the best decisions for all individuals, as authorities often make speculative and wrong judgments on facts and science, sometimes flip-flopping on answers to cover their tracks in some weird action of covering their ignorance of facts. No authority has all the answers. There are many individuals that have many answers, and it is appropriate such individuals form factions and declare changes to a flawed Vaccine Act and flawed vaccine programs that fail in addressing vaccine safety. I have read about and talked to many individuals that would agree to the need to fix flaws in the Vaccine Act. I however would suggest such actions are a waste of time. The Vaccine Act has outlived its short-term purpose, which was to give vaccine manufacturers an unplanned safety net relating to vaccine-injury liability. This protection is no longer needed, and the safety net provided to manufacturers and medical professionals should have been short-term. The Vaccine Act does not make healthcare better or vaccines safer but makes vaccines safety more discretionary and a greater threat of harm to citizens.

The Vaccine Act has pushed a law which mandates acceptance of a "no harm, no foul, and all parties must agree the injured individuals simply goes away with a small sum of money to stay silent" settlement, which is a standard practice among insurance companies and attorneys attempting to facilitate a quick settlement which they suggest benefits all parties, but generally does not benefit the injured party. Children are often further discounted as noncitizens and non-wage earners compared to their needs and value to society in these types of settlements. What you may ask is the point of vaccinating? The arguments for many vaccines are quite weak. Yet, Vaccine Inc parties gladly go along and promote CDC guidelines and recommendations. Authorities suggest citizens should accept vaccine injuries as oddities as everyone knows bizarre science happens all the time. Authorities suggest there is no reason to pay attention to case reports of vaccine-related injuries, or even science that explain mechanisms of causation. The main point for vaccination is protection of oneself, not safety from adverse harms.

Individuals can make the greatest impact as factional groups of influencers that demand our government fully address adverse vaccine injuries before offering false promotions that vaccines are safe. Take away the promotional backing, and vaccines will find fewer supporters, as medical professionals and manufacturers will also be required to address vaccine-related injuries and liability. The cost for all Vaccine Inc parties in the vaccine business will explode, but maybe they should explode to help citizens find a better and fairer line in the sand for vaccine safety, if such safety is even possible. Better infectious disease therapeutic treatment protocols, health care resources and training, and infectious disease educational measures are better options for addressing both drug and public safety.

Citizens can affect these changes through several meaningful actions. Terminating the Vaccine Act and the VICP would be the proper first step to force Vaccine Inc to address the need for vaccine safety, and eliminate false promotional standards for vaccines as being suggestively safe drugs. Regulation and oversight are mandated in many health and drug laws but are overlooked as a favor to many commercial interests. Science and medical professionals are constrained in their ability to perform their job duties if authorities do not supply correct and transparent facts and data to make proper professional judgements first. Authorities often shift their private failures as justification for making discretionary actions the preferred action in laws, taking away individuals rights rather than empowering individuals with facts and science.

I suggest individuals must band together as factions of concerned citizens who demand we address the Vaccine Law as a serious safety concern for citizens. Our government cannot promote, advocate, and spend endlessly on vaccines, if the public simply rejects many vaccines which are not as impactful today as they once were, without addressing both adverse safety concerns and effectiveness at the outset of approval, and such concerns must be continually addressed as ongoing safety concerns.

Authorities should be concerned about plagues, pandemics, and other epidemiologic outbreaks, but the questions asked should be scientific based and directed through a more open public discussion where facts and science are easily accessible. Citizens should help each other understand or have access to healthcare professionals that can provide accurate information in informing citizens of facts and science, and not directing citizens to poorly trained government phone representatives that read from a script, which is promotional, and not informative. I suggest this will not happen without also impacting the government's bottom line (or some would say profit) on vaccines, which as I stated before our government "is all in" on vaccines. If money is an addiction, our government is clearly hooked on vaccines as a financial tool. Citizens need public service announcements to be informative, whereas most government guidance and recommendations are misguided and unhelpful. Citizens cannot expect our government to change its ways overnight, or even over decades.

As a medical professional, I began my research of vaccines going back several decades ago, as I have remained informed regarding risks and providing proper counselling, even as it was not commonly part of a pharmacist's duties to administer vaccines until around 2008. The professional transition for many pharmacists was not smooth, but it was also clear many doctors did not always want to vaccinate patients either, generally deferring duties to a nurse or other trained agent of the doctor. Believe it or not, some highly trained medical professionals simply dislike needles and fear the vaccine injuries or their poor skills in administering the vaccine may cause an injury, which is oddly in some manner lessened as a fear if they did not personally administer the vaccine.

Again, all medical professionals should fully understand that vaccine injuries can occur with all vaccines, but many parties do not care to expand on vaccine injury discussions, as they will often defer to CDC guidelines and statements as their government-endorsed professional reference for need and safety. Many medical professionals suggest sufficient data and evidence of safety exists for vaccines, I suggest all drugs and vaccines fall under drug laws which prohibit hiding risks and safety concerns "in any particular". Meaning it is against the law in every state and in federal drug laws to hide and fail to address a drug adverse safety concern, but vaccines are given a free pass, which I find unacceptable. I do find it interesting several COVID-19 vaccine manufacturers are taking a firm stance on safety concerns yet I still have my doubts safety concerns are being addressed as vaccine manufacturers will roll out a COVID-19 vaccine approved under discretionary emergency approval with limited adverse concerns addressed, perhaps pointing to a more comprehensive plan to address such adverse events related to the vaccine in the future. Again, limited vaccine liability leads to marginal changes and actions as soon as the vaccine is approved and released to the mass market. The FDA's approval for mass marketing of a vaccine is the key to granting release of vaccine liability to the VICP.

The FDA does not have to address all vaccine concerns for post-marketing adverse drug events for years, or even decades. The VICP and HHS likewise can also take years or decades to address an injury concern. I personally would reject any vaccine manufacturer's claim of addressing a safety concerns as a vaccine being pushed through clinical trials in rapid fashion which cannot possibly address large-scale reporting of vaccine-related injuries that can take months or longer to be found and understood. Vaccine injuries are simply poorly reported adverse events before, during and after FDA approval. The manufacturers and the FDA know the game. The game has been played for decades now, and our government thinks the public is unwise to the game. Vaccine injury promotional management is a game created by and administered by our government. Vaccine manufacturers silently playing the game alongside the government. I do not play along with Vaccine Inc but demand better tools, data, and information, and reject the need for vaccines where a vaccine is not needed as the best or only drug treatment option.

A medical professional's idea of unacceptable, is another citizen's definition of being perfectly okay. As some people say, what you do with your body is your choice. You can decide what is best for your body, but if you are a parent you are deciding for a child who has no understanding of facts and drug safety issues. For that, your child will count on you. Just consider my statements as "fair warning" and you have now been given fair warning. All vaccines certainly can cause adverse drug reactions and injuries, and the injuries are not fully addressed by our government or medical professionals.

Drug reporting is always ongoing; before, during and after a drug is approved. Generally, under a discretionary good faith effort that the FDA did the best job it could in an allotted timeframe. Often by the same authorities who issue approvals and guidelines and government funding, then reverse course after reevaluating the data months or years later. Authorities often shift course, but only at the risk of a public shaming. As fair reference, I have seen product information statements submitted to the FDA grow from a few pages to being over 50+ pages of safety and adverse concerns in less than a decade. This kind of rapid increase in a safety profile would imply the FDA is often less restrictive on the front end of approval of many drugs but demands more data as length of time a drug is on the market passes. COVID-19 is receiving exceptional discretion, which I will simply state warrants exceptional caution. Whereas many other novel vaccines, which are generally novel therapeutic vaccines, move slower through clinical trials and provide more safety and effectiveness data before being approved. Again, I simply restate, the COVID-19 vaccine calls for proper caution and demands exceptional data and safety review before being accepted by citizens as safe.

Many citizens object to the FDA's discretionary behavior, as the FDA is mandated to supply complete drug information to the public. The FDA facts and other federal agencies regulatory actions often supply confusing information to the public, and often even confuse doctors, who are not pharmacists, and do not fully understand some pharmacological actions relating to many drugs, including basic warnings and adverse drug reactions. Drug safety profiles can be a bit too much for them to grasp or they do not have the time to review the details which can be too much to process without further details and references.

Not that I am perfect or review every detail from the manufacturer or FDA statements down to smallest adverse reaction but if it is reported somewhere to a manufacturer who must review and report noted concerns and when there is evidence of an adverse drug reactions, such adverse reactions are simply waiting to be researched and understood. This is the position of the National Academy of Science, but not the FDA or other government agencies, as government authorities often take a more wait and see approach before acting. And some noted drug-related injuries are held back for years on a wait and see basis, before being added to the product information statements. Drug product information statements are available online, or simply ask a pharmacist or doctor to print a product information statement for you, if you have questions about any drug. The product information statement can be a large printout, but always ask for the Brand Name Product Information (PI) statement, as generic companies generally have limited drug information reporting requirements. For the most complete information, select the professional prescriber complete disclosure statement if given a choice. This is the most complete approved public drug record readily accessible to the public.

I state my concerns for many vaccines and especially influenza and COVID vaccines not as an outsider, but as an informed insider. I have made many phone calls, letters, emails, and other forms of communications to high ranking, often the highest-level, public authorities who often limit their access to the public. A few authorities are sincere, where sincerity is good, but supply some implied morality favoring vaccine benefits which does not address an adverse vaccine reaction. Simple full public disclosure of facts reported in post-marketing data and case reports would be useful to many citizens and medical professionals. The FDA and many government agencies complain, and state "we ain't got no money" to provide complete vaccine data and facts. For which I would state if you cannot do your job as stated in drug laws, maybe there is only limited need for the agency, which is a conclusion many medical professionals accept as being the current standards of government regulation and enforcement practices used every day. Perhaps all citizens should understand our government pours hundreds of billions of dollars into failing healthcare regulatory programs every year.

I have filed complaints (called a Citizen's Petition) for vaccine-related injuries to the FDA. Only to see the first complaint shuffled to low level staff. Yet a citizen can follow the path of a complaint with added FOIA requests if a citizen really wants to try an extended route for resolution. I believe the FDA and other authorities like this route, as they hope the citizen will eventually just give up and walk away in disgust. Citizens can find out who last held the complaint, but this is not an answer, as a citizen can call that individual and they will simply pass it to another staffer, most likely one with no authority to do anything. Keep this up and you will speak to dozens of FDA staff members in the vaccine safety department, but never get anything resolved. I learned long ago how to skip over useless staffers in government agencies, but the process requires a little effort and finesse, as authorities often have gatekeepers to keep out unwanted citizens. Again, addressing vaccine safety concerns are a transparency issue which has been shuffled, underfunded, and rarely addressed.

I suggest citizens bypass this mess, by simply call the highest-ranking doctors in charge of drug safety and vaccine safety and ask them directly to address the safety concern. And again, spend hours in talks with them, where they agree to forward the concerns to an appropriate workgroup of medical professionals (who are maintained secretly away from public and even medical professional cannot be given their names), and will promise to get back with you ASAP. This is the most common game all authorities at the FDA play, as I have made the calls, and I have documented the discussions, some hours long in discussions with high level medical experts, or at least the ones that eventually answer their phones. Citizens may ask who are these authorities? Most of the authorities are physicians, as pharmacists do not seem qualified to run a federal drug program or agency or even drug review department, even though pharmacists also carry the title of doctors and understand the drug benefits and risks better. Many FDA employed pharmacists agree with my concerns for vaccine-related injury reporting, but cannot say so to their bosses, as that might cost them their jobs, which are typically lower on the FDA totem pole.

Many authorities also have political or prior industry experience and aspirations. A few authorities are simply glad to work in a government job, and many enjoy the power and prestige that presumably goes with their positions. The lines between a citizen's concerns and an administrative or regulatory concern are often very gray areas of concern. Suggesting the authority must move it to the next level of authority to get a yes or no answer before answering a concern as most officials operate with limited oversight or recourse for lack of skills or knowledge of the facts. A complex issue or concern can take years to work up the ladder of officials, unless a citizen takes shortcuts, which are not obvious, but are available.

I would hope a mandatory change in vaccine regulatory and/or drug laws will be inevitable some day in the future. Hopefully, one day, my suggested public actions are heard and demanded as actions the public mandates as being needed to be addressed as valid concerns. Citizens can and should take the time and take important steps in advocating for public safety and vaccine drug safety, which are mutually inclusive actions. Authorities often do not even attempt to keep up with large volumes of information or cannot keep up with the science or drug review requirements, and citizens often elect foolish politicians who appoint foolish staff who operate behind closed doors and not in the public's best interests, but often in their self-interests.

Politicians always say they love our country, but actions speak loader than words, and should be more meaningful if you make a campaign promise to address concerns and do not follow through to even take minor steps to address the concerns promised would be addressed while campaigning. Politicians clearly like to flip-flop on the issue of vaccines, expressing their concerns about vaccine-related injuries then suggesting there are no concerns for injuries at all, and suggest that vaccines are the best and safest options available for citizens. This perhaps being an educational instructive manipulation technique they teach students at the University of Pennsylvania, as their graduates often use the flip-flop statements for political and business purposes. Suggest honest concerns, then flip on the answer when asked later why the concerns are now different. Are citizens stupid? At UPenn and other elite schools they are taught to act as if they are smarter, and that there is a need to cast aside the doubts and concerns of simple citizens. True answers however are in science, which authorities and Noble Liars often forget to consider before talking philosophically. Citizens can and must demand the need for added vaccine science and citizens do not need an intellectual elitist to look the science up. Citizens can look the science up themselves. Our government authorities should simply make the information easier to find. If you have a question on my facts and methods for contacting the proper authorities, simply ask, and I will try to get to your requests as soon as possible. Again, my website is www.VNTY.Health.

CHAPTER 10

The Citizen's Responsibility

Is It IDK (I Don't Know) or IDC (I Don't Care)?

'If you wish to strive for peace of soul and pleasure, then believe; if you wish to be a devotee of truth, then inquire". Friedrich Nietzsche

Citizens often claim to know or understand drug risks, but rather than inquire about facts they simply believe what they are told as the truth. A simple outlook on life which generally requires little insight or investigation. A commitment to truth, justice and fairness are qualities that separate us as citizens and separates us as nations. Truth is a matchless quality which sets us apart. Accepting responses of IDK or IDC are measures of believing and trusting authorities that have not earned a citizen's trust. It is also the first sign of individuals playing the stupid card. The cards one plays when they do not know the answers or possible outcome but hope to play out the game and win. The VICP and many Vaccine Inc players love to play this type of game, because they manipulate and control the cards, we must use to play the game.

Citizens play nonsensical games all the time, as do authorities; but it is important to understand that citizens must inquire and ask questions. And not just for oneself but also for your loved ones and those you care about the most. I made deep dive inquiries on many facts about causation of a vaccine injury, and the subsequent medical complications. I could have stopped and trusted and believed some very highly trained and knowledgeable experts would take appropriate actions, but instead continued to inquire and learned for myself, as a medical professional, to help my loved one.

I researched many nephrotic cases and studied which cases and studies proved relapses of nephrotic syndrome as being triggered by vaccines. Many nephrologists conceding an understanding of the well-known complication but often gave idiopathic answers, like, "they did not know what specific mechanisms caused a nephrotic relapse" or "they did not care to do the research" to investigate the issue, as the drug mechanism analysis was "too complex". As the medical difficulties for my son's vaccine injury case progressed, I experienced another round of IDKs or IDCs. And treating specialists simply vanished from the scene and stopped signing medical records, referring treatments to be addressed by a nurse. Medical records grew sketchy, and a change in the treating specialist was mandated. A change in drug treatment resulted in some success but did not fully stabilize the nephrotic relapse following the flu vaccine, which relapsed again when taken off the lesser documented immunosuppressing drug which subsequently led to further immune and vascular complications.

I researched the source for the cause of the complications and found numerous case reports and studies were related to a treatment protocol which I tracked back to being a vaccine-related injury. Influenza vaccines are a noted source of triggering a nephrotic condition in many patients. The flu vaccine can also trigger a sequence of nephrotic medical complications which can lead to further exacerbation of the nephrotic state. Medical complications can become extraordinarily complex. A worsening of a pre-existing medical condition the Vaccine Act states is covered as a vaccine-related injury, as the exacerbation was not stabilized for over 1 year. To stabilize the complicated relapse, my son was put on a different immunosuppressing class of drugs called calcineurin inhibitors (or CNIs). The drug was Prograf which helped manage the nephrotic state but led to vascular issues that caused a cerebrovascular stroke injury known as atypical PRES (posterior reversible encephalopathy syndrome). These extremely serious complicating adverse events related to Prograf could have been addressed earlier if the manufacturer, Astellas, had simply addressed the adverse drug reactions when the ADR was discovered in 1996, but again we run into a different set of IDK and IDC responses by disinterested parties.

PRES was outlined as a Prograf drug warning, but the FDA and Astellas did not fully report facts of the ADR until 2013. Today, PRES is a documented and recognized risk tied to cerebrovascular events through an atypical development of inflammation and vascular injury complications in arteries that supply blood to the brain, but again about 20 years after the facts were originally discovered and reported in the New England Journal of Medicine. But in 2010, my son began taking Prograf with no risk of PRES being reported in low doses he would be taking to manage his nephrotic condition. Astellas and the FDA inadequately listed the concern in its approved drug statements, and the manufacturer even denied the concern in 2011 when I contacted their pharmacovigilant team for more information. Astellas however changed its position in 2012 with a change in listed manufacturer concern by issuing an Important Safety Information drug warning guidance statement for Prograf in 2013. Again, today all medical professionals should understand the serious adverse risks of Prograf and other CNIs when used to treat nephrotic patients.

Prograf was the true source of my son's most significant future medical complications relating to a treatment plan which became mandatory after standard protocols failed to stabilize his condition following the vaccine-induced nephrotic relapse injury. If this sound too complicated it probably is for most citizens and even for most medical professionals, but the Vaccine Act states this type of exacerbated medical complication sequence is covered under the VICP, as the vaccine clearly started the sequence and prolonged treatment with drugs that have less well-understood safety profiles which were required in an attempt to find balance but instead created more complications which are worse, defined in the Vaccine Act as an exacerbation of a pre-existing medical condition.

I point this out, as my son's vaccine injury is not the simple and straightforward adverse vaccine reaction. In fact, it is extraordinarily complex. Initially, I considered Prograf as the primary drug liability component, but after discussing the issue with the VICP attorney and our nephrology doctor, both agreed the vaccine-related injury was the beginning drug factor and it was a covered injury listed in the Vaccine Law. In fact, the VICP special master even agreed to the argument in the first meeting following a filing of the claim in 2012. Why argue the complex Prograf adverse reaction when the VICP special master already accepted the vaccine injury claim, in 2012? And again, in 2013. And in 2016. And even in 2017.

The Vaccine Act however is not just a single failure, but a double failure for my son. The Vaccine Injury Compensation Program's special master does not need to understand facts and vaccines mechanisms well, but can randomly agree to the claim facts as worthy of being settled for over 5 years, then change their mind. The VICP is an odd federal reconciliation court program. Most medical and pharmaceutical liability cases are based on state laws and are settled in state courts. Vaccine and drug liability cases are two completely different set of laws, and there are zero lawyers that effectively understand both arguments. In fact, many state-based lawyers have stated a drug lawsuit would be difficult to present to a jury as a jury would likely point to the vaccine as being the cause of the injury. Even as the federal Courts took over 7 years to fully address the vaccine injury claim, wrongly deciding the vaccine was not related to the most serious complication, in the shockingly bad impulsive opinion of a special master and other judges who have no understanding of drug mechanisms, cruelly resorting to twisting medical records and ignoring arguments on science and facts previously accepted to craft their flawed legal opinions.

One would think my son's injury was a perfect example of a straightforward pharmaceutical liability lawsuit, but it is not, as lawyers do not know how the science works and did not care to inquire. Ms. Millman, the VICP special master, said she understood the medical complication and recommended settlement in 2012 and again during the five years that followed. Dr. Bellanti covered Prograf in his 2013 expert letter to the VICP court. A collection of drug facts which were stated as understood by all parties. But then Drs. Kaplan and Levinson, the government's experts, played the stupid card in 2017 during the trial.

Encouraged by the DOJ attorneys and Ms. Millman, both government experts alleged they did not believe my son's treatment protocols could cause such a complication, which was either a pure lack of drug expertise or perhaps both were fully out-of-date on current Prograf drug facts. Again, the warning is listed in the current Prograf manufacturer product information statement, so I am not sure how anyone could miss the warning statement, but again drug experts are not permitted to discuss pharmaceutical facts in a VICP hearing. Only a limited number of hired and biased physicians can talk about the vaccine injury and drug science. And to add to the problems, the special master can decide to condense and cut a full discussion of drug injury-related mechanisms in a VICP trial hearing. Who knew such a highly positioned federal court could be so biased and cruel?

The special master told our experts she understood the facts, then apparently decided the Prograf facts no longer mattered in her limited vaccine-specific legal world. Sudden acts of ignorance and misunderstanding of drug facts by several self-proclaimed medical and legal experts is inexcusable. I say it is certain, the influenza vaccine triggered the sudden relapse, as nothing else likely could have caused the relapse. It fits the FDA definition of an Adverse Drug Reaction (ADR) perfectly. The relapse became more complicated, requiring a shift in treatment to Prograf. The Prograf caused serious medical complications including PRES and multiple cerebral strokes. These are all noted medical facts, and by law covered by the Vaccine Act. Ms. Millman and the government however shifted facts, which one would think is illegal, and changed earlier statements I made, which one would think of as inappropriate. If they wanted to change facts, they should have sought to dismiss the case in 2012, and not dragged it out until 2017. Perhaps, making a

Prograf liability case easier to pursue where a lawyer could have understood the Prograf complications better without all of Ms. Millman's nonsense interpretations of science and facts. I simply say shame on Ms. Millman, Dr. Kaplan, and the other government parties for not knowing the facts, for changing the facts to fit a false narrative, and for harming a child. All government parties fitting the definition of being pathic human beings.

I could end the argument here, but given it took over 8 years to address the VICP court process, my son's only option for legal remedy would fall to him to seek remedy as he officially became an adult, a citizen, and my role shifted to being a supportive care person, which is like a guardian but does not have the same legal rights for legal representation. Both legal cases were forced on a disabled adult with limited communicative skills, to an exceptionally poor state legal system that does not adequately address legal cases for disabled people with communications disabilities. I found many state-based lawyers are unfamiliar with vaccine laws, and the majority of attorneys are unwilling to address drug cases that are not class action cases, as costs to litigate an injury to a single child/adult is too high for a case against a manufacturer that is part of a multi-trillion-dollar conglomerate. Vaccines, stupidity, and lack of interest are the ultimate IDK and IDC ideologies for attorneys.

Personally, I passionately believe the VICP program and Ms. Millman deliberately harmed my son, and his case which sought a legitimate vaccine injury settlement. Not as it relates to a vaccine-related injury, but because Ms. Millman and the DOJ had created some invisible cap on claim costs, where neither Ms. Millman or the

DOJ's pack of vaccine-committed attorneys did not care to address the costs of my son's medical experts-determined injury damage cost estimates, which were meticulously determined by medical professionals in the marketplace, and the government's authorities clearly cannot properly address scientific and medical facts. Ms. Millman and Mr. Wishard dismissed facts and did not allow discussion of science facts that are stated in black and white which are inexcusable actions in almost every profession. Yet the VICP and federal courts consider such actions okay and acceptable when the matter involves vaccines and vaccine-related injuries.

Unfortunately, I have heard the word "I don't care" enough, to quickly tell the stupid attorneys, I DO care, and I know enough other people that care that I have no plans to ever give up on understanding an obvious vaccine-related injury and medical facts. A vaccine injury case for any individual should never be dismissed as being inconsequential to our government authorities that originally made the false promise to all citizens to address vaccine-related injuries when the injury facts are clear. Multiple parties today, including lawyers and federal agencies clearly have developed an aversion to vaccine-related cases, as they simply slither away from any case that has to do with vaccines. I absolutely do care and would be happy to help individuals with drug facts, but injured parties must understand lawsuits at both the federal and state level are time sensitive and the federal Courts and VICP harm a citizen's right to address the injuries in state courts, as both have statutes of limitation relating to a narrow timeframe to file a lawsuit.

Citizen might think the doctors surely know the injury and vaccine facts, and can help correct an injustice, but most doctors hate the court system, and are taught from the first year of medical school not to get involved. Right after taking the Hippocratic Oath pledging to protect all patients, they get the lessons on how to avoid being involved in lawsuits. And doctors prefer to stick to their clinical practices rather than dig into mechanisms of drug actions and various mechanisms of causation of an injury. All federal Courts address vaccine-related concerns following the IDC and IDK standards of practice and policies. Vaccines cases are awkward and disrespectful. The VICP has been chosen by our government as being the sole court to address vaccine-related injuries, and the VICP special masters' opinions are outrageously discretionary. Medical facts, records, and evidence are shamefully reviewed using outrageous discretion. Not only medical arguments, but arguments shaped to fit a narrative and to fit a final predetermined conclusion, which is often harshly flawed in its interpretation of science and medical facts.

Citizens should be very skeptical of any court that offers such a dangerous combination of discretion, manipulation, and outright prohibition of discussions of vaccine scientific facts. Accurate and clear medical records can help an argument, but good luck finding multiple doctors who can help and have also kept good medical records. The standards of medical recordkeeping in our medical system are shockingly bad and pulling records together even when you know what records should be present are extremely challenging. And finding multiple experts in medicine, rehabilitation, finance, arbitration, and life care planning are also difficult areas to address. These are all huge tasks, but maybe you can do better, in the wicked and false VICP injury claims program, if you should ever choose to file a claim seeking settlement of a vaccine injury. Remember, it is not a lawsuit against a vaccine manufacturer for an injury the vaccine triggered, but a claim against the vaccine drug which our government promised to protect and limit claims against the vaccine class of drugs. I cannot imagine any citizen having much better luck in the government-endorsed and created VICP. So again, take the risk at your own discretion, but do not say you have not been warned. The nonsense our government uses to oversee the Vaccine Act is scary stupid, both legally and medically, using scientific and legal arguments few citizens could follow as being valid or logical. I do care about vaccine injuries, but I have found few other parties that care about vaccine-related injuries, and fewer that understand mechanisms of vaccine-related injury which could one day impact many patients that simply did not care to inquire and learn about our flawed Vaccine Law and VICP.

I would love to believe our government cares, but considering how much the Noble Liars lie by saying they care about all citizens, and that individuals can trust them, but the reality is the government only wants to make you believe they can be trusted, and that they quietly enacted a vaccine law which has become an evil administrative tool for determining vaccine injuries which citizens cannot trust. Citizens should not trust our government, and should not trust our courts relating to vaccine concerns, or vaccine manufacturers who have little interest in addressing vaccine injuries, and the medical professionals who are also protected from liability claims and willingly go along with the promotional vaccine statements, while also failing to address vaccine injuries occurring in their medical practice.

Citizens want a higher level of trust from these parties, but the trust is invalidated when the parties also freely make IDK and IDC discretionary statements and ignore testimony and discussion of valid reported science. Citizens must demand full access to vaccine information including all reported adverse vaccine reactions, which now must be done independently of our government, as our government often hides these facts from both citizens and medical professionals.

All physicians and pharmacists are licensed medical professionals in the states where they work and take care of patients. It is the medical professional's legal duty to address all inquiries by patients seeking medical facts and vital information needed to make informed decisions for their health. While there are plenty of IDK or IDC opportunities, as medical professionals often do not want to admit to their lack of training and expertise, and may state, "I don't know" when pressed for a fact, but should also supplement the IDK with "I will try to find out an answer for you" with a promise to get back with you ASAP with answers. These answers often save lives or improves a patient's medical condition or recovery. It is an endless pursuit to help others solve their health concerns. All medical professionals are not so helpful, and many offer guidance and recommendations that sound more like IDK or IDC answers. Vaccine injuries and answers to citizens' concerns will never be answered by IDK and IDC type answers. Citizens can be disappointed in all parties that state little understanding of vaccines, yet openly advertise and promote the need for vaccines. I reject these government and medical parties' claims for a need for vaccines on a regular basis.

I suggest citizens commit to making in-depth inquires of all vaccines, and demand reasonable scientific information to make fair and informed decisions, knowing the answers are now available and our government and many medical professionals do not care to address or provide in-depth information about vaccine injuries. The art of nondisclosure and oversimplification of vaccine benefits and injury statements have been lowered to statements that are dumb-down vaccine fact statements. Individuals must look to inquire about facts and demand transparency and change, not just for themselves but for citizens that cannot make such informed decisions for themselves. I inquired about vaccine-related facts not just for my son, but for all individuals that are harmed and injured by vaccines. Some vaccines are clearly a source for serious medical problems, and the vaccine-related injuries are poorly addressed and reported. Influenza vaccines have more VICP injury claims than many other vaccines combined. The injuries are not listed on the Vaccine Injury Table and the DOJ will uncompromisingly refuse to settle off-Table injuries, which results in unresolved fact-based injuries and no reasonable options to resolve the claim, which again is not what the government promised citizens when enacting the Vaccine Act in 1986.

The VICP program puts individuals attempting to claim injuries at an immediate disadvantage to resolve a claim, and immediately permits open bias against the claim, with statements often expressed as IDK or IDC, and demand acceptance of a marginal settlement and demand full release of vaccine liability being the cause of the injury or exacerbated medical complications. Where Vaccine Inc often uses a false statement of caring and knowledge of medical facts which are not true, which I can validate the VICP and Vaccine Inc are in fact the worst offenders of both IDK and IDC.

Transparency and accessibility to data and facts, and open discussions are critical to showing scientific truths. I suggest transparency should follow the acronym KISS, which is a belief that all rules and laws must **K**eep **I**t **S**imple **S**ir (or Stupid depending on the situation). KISS can fall down a slippery slope of IDK and IDC and given discretion over extended periods where facts and laws become less simple and exclusionary. The government enacted the Vaccine Act with promised KISS-like actions but have failed to deliver simplicity and transparency to citizens. The Vaccine Act and our government have failed to address vaccine injuries and adverse vaccine reactions to simplify our lives and our understanding of medical and drug facts, and openly promote the perverse law as a solution for addressing vaccine-related injuries affecting both children and adults.

These actions by multiple parties do not use science or facts but often use the ASSUME stamp of approval made in the best interests of uninformed citizens. But as I learned long ago, it is never right to ASSUME anything about facts even where the facts are available right in a person's face. For I learned long ago, if you ASS/U/ME anything and do not have the facts, it will make an ass out of U and ME, and who wants to be an ASS. Our government clearly does not mind, because that is all our government does in making decisions on a regular basis. Assume they know more than the citizens, then decide what they will do and what the citizens must do, because they decided it was the best thing for all citizens to do. Forgetting most citizens do not like assumptions and random discretions.

Most citizens prefer to keep it simple, keep it transparent, and make the facts and laws accessible for discussion. Our Constitution mandates these decision-making principles. Where fair and just jury trials are heard by citizens who are peers that will hear full facts and arguments, not granting full discretionary decisions to a single special master playing a game of sophistication and flawed science.

Again, we must punctuate the individual's voice, as the individual makes the final decisions in how they chose to live their lives. The power to inquire is an extraordinarily strong tool to learn, but the right to inquire is also a right a citizen can easily overlook. Our government assumes citizens will overlook this right, and further assumes our government's authorities can make the decisions and recommendations for all citizens. This however is the wrong assumption for many citizens who demand more facts and science in our justice system.

The Vaccine Act and the VICP program are not what the government promised when they enacted the Vaccine Act as a vaccine manufacturer and medical profession liability protection law. Lawyers develop "assume-based" arguments which lead to illogical bad discretionary legal concepts and applications. Doctors in their medical practice will use science developed as understandings of laws of nature and medicine. And if either side becomes sidetracked by IDK or IDC arguments, the parties rarely seek out a more knowledgeable independent party. The special master is not an independent party by any valid definition of independence. The VICP program is a legal resolution program that falsely offers a discretionary outcome based on opinions, not science understood by a single special master, over an extended period of time. A program where doctors do not know or understand the Vaccine Law, and lawyers do not fully know the medicine or science. And citizens are simply left out of the discussion as statements are made showing a lack of caring and because of the legal parties' endless need for assumptions. I call the VICP courtroom, stupid courtroom science drama, where legal and medical experts are happy to act as sham experts, forgetting a child was injured and a legal promise was made to address a notable and documented vaccine-related injury.

So many principles of law are either ignored or abused in the VICP court, it would make an average citizen's head spin in disbelief. Forget government experts that lie and perjure themselves, which is considered perfectly acceptable. The Department of Justice practices a harmful, hateful form of big-bully government defense law, which might be acceptable in a normal courtroom where parties are arguing extremely antagonistic arguments to persuade a jury which party is correct, but the VICP's form of legal arguments was not how the Vaccine Act was set up to address vaccine injuries. The VICP does not need to untwist facts into something less understood; but must address the facts so the citizens can understand the law, and at some point limit harm to individuals. The VICP however twists science to fit their conclusions and Vaccine Act allows special master to make false "independent" opinions, which are not informative, and is harmful to both citizens and science. Science and vaccine facts are left unanswered and few parties in our government care to address these important vaccine drug concerns.

Many citizens may state IDK or IDC to these VICP court decisions and government actions relating to vaccines, but as citizens of a society with laws designated as protection of citizen rights and giving individuals the power to make choices, we must care, and we must become knowledgeable of foolish laws and how these laws are dealt with for individuals and by individuals. The government does not have to care and does not have to address our concerns. Citizens must find alternative methods of addressing our concerns. And that includes making every effort to force our government to be transparent and to allow citizens the opportunity to be vocal in their concerns.

If we simply grant these false decisions by authorities as being acceptable, then we as citizens will be rejecting our rights to inquire, and by extension our rights to make a choice. Hoping and believing someone is making the right choices for us. Citizens must understand they will be trusting authorities who will do as they wish, not what is right or should be properly addressed in an open forum. IDK and IDC are important concerns that highlight a power-grab by authorities at individual rights protected under our constitution. It is our duty as citizens to mandate our inquiries must be addressed and seek out discoveries to address our concerns relating to vaccine injuries through truths and science, and not through discretionary opinions and authoritative beliefs.

CHAPTER 11

What Forums are Available to Advocate for Citizen Rights?

Citizens today must consider all actions of how drugs work in the body before they accept the recommendations of our government and in many cases the recommendations of their healthcare professionals. Each drug recommendation often comes with a list of benefits of usage but also require a discussion of adverse drug reactions and warnings. And an even longer list of potential adverse drug reactions exists which are generally poorly reported or addressed and are often left out of the opening discussion. Vaccine manufacturers offer poorly reported adverse injury data for many vaccines, and our government offers self-reporting and voluntary reporting of vaccine injuries by individuals and healthcare providers as part of their solution to vaccine adverse safety concerns. One system is bad, and the other system is insanely bad. The need for a forum to discuss such vaccine drug details is great, as our government shrinks in its duty and passes on important discussions which must be addressed to provide science and fairness to a law designed to save a class of drugs, vaccines.

As a citizen considers vaccines, first consider that vaccines are drugs, specifically known as dangerous drugs. Dangerous drug with limited avenues for redress if an adverse drug reaction should occur. Do citizens understand the Vaccine Act? Legally known as the National Childhood Vaccine Injury Act of 1986. Citizens often have no idea what rights are granted or taken away as they relate to informed consent laws, where the individual has the right to demand information and be informed of risks and benefits for all drugs, including vaccines. A CDC Vaccine Information Statement is a recommended substitute for a more detailed drug product information sheet, as citizens are given the right to be counselled "in the moment" to demand additional vaccine details and facts before a vaccination. And if a citizen has questions, ask about how the vaccine programs and the VICP works. Citizens should inquire about as much information as necessary to be comfortable in giving up rights granted to inquire, or perhaps the future need to file a vaccine injury claim in our nation's only vaccine court of law, as well as addressing all adverse vaccine reaction information stated and understood in medical literature.

Citizens must understand the Vaccine Act and injury compensation programs are narrow, limited legal actions; and the programs are administered as authoritarian autocracies with special masters and reviewing judges, in place of a time-honored constitutional-mandated jury. One should remember juries, as juries are needed for fairness under the constitution, but juries have been legislated as unnecessary for citizens by our government relating to a commercial set of drugs. Perhaps, citizens could get a fair reference, if they work for a large company, and the head of human resources were suddenly given total authority through a law to address workers compensation claims as they see fit, without any actual competency granted to address the injury concern through any other legal remedy. This type of law did happen in the Industrial Age of the 1800s, where commercial big businesses controlled or held influence over many government actions and interests, with financial payoffs and harmful combined financial interests.

For decades, child labor laws and other adverse working conditions were perfectly okay with our government, even encouraged in some businesses. The VICP program is that awful, causing harm to selected parties, and our government never even making a real effort to address the vaccine safety concerns. Maybe worse than awful, since the program often drags out a vaccine injury claim for years, and the claim is often made for the benefit of a child. These government and vaccine industry oversight parties are greedy, heartless little people. The VICP is that bad as special masters often decide cases with a slanted bias in favor of Vaccine Inc, which the government wholeheartedly represents and promotes as partners in public health. The special masters are attorneys with no exceptional medical training, some with about the same level of scientific intelligence of a human resource manager. So, without question, citizens should be very wary of our Vaccine Injury Compensation Program.

These are issues citizens must ponder with vaccines. What are the vaccine drug's mechanisms of action and mechanisms of causation relating to an adverse reaction, and what injuries are possible and reported as being vaccine-related by scientists hoping to address vaccine injuries? What are the risks to oneself if a vaccine is skipped? And is the infectious disease really that big of a concern, based on the individual's age and current lifestyle and living arrangement? What are the alternatives to vaccines if a citizen were to skip the vaccine? Again, is the vaccine necessary? Who are the advocates (Doctors? It must be a physician!) for an individual if the individual is injured, for medical treatments and for a VICP claims? Does the government offer a fair and transparent forum to learn as much as possible, before, during or after a vaccination? The answers and the suggested government forums are pathetically insufficient. Again with a lot of dumbed-down statements and promotional information, and if citizens want to participate in any government forum, they are given a small window to make a public statement, and if you are really ambitious you can file a Citizen's Petition demanding action by the FDA. Not that any such action will result in any government action, but at least you will know where you stand in relationship to vaccines and our government, which is exceptionally low on their concerns list. Vaccines are exceptionally high on their most valued drugs list. One could almost call our government a bunch of vaccine junkies.

When the Vaccine Act was passed in 1986, our government made promises to citizens it knew immediately could not be kept, which was fair and proper care of all citizens and especially children injured by the vaccines. Promise a lot (protection, new therapeutics, impartial and fair-minded concerns for injured patients) and deliver a little (missing safety reporting, promotional statements, and misguided judges), which sounds like an exceptionally bad business plan; but a bad business plan we fund as taxpayers and end-users of the commercial vaccine product every year. Costs continually rise, but the funding source stays the same, and mandatory payout limits and settlements are frozen from 35 years ago. Nobody in the VICP has apparently heard of the word inflation, as health care costs have grown at a rate substantially higher than the overall economy, but the costs paid out to experts and attorneys continually grows at the current rate of inflation or higher. Does this sound like a good business model for citizens to you? Sounds like a failed business model to me. At some point the business "squeeze" must happen, and the party in the squeeze to limit settlement are the citizens who are injured. The citizens are suggestively thought to be stupid and will accept welfare as a path to resolve a vaccine-related injury, while our vaccine authorities live comfortable and well-paid and in many cases over-paid lives.

Vaccine Inc has centralized and federalized vaccine safety research functions over the last few decades. The CDC partners with the American Medical Association and its provincial organizations like the American Pediatric Association, to develop selling strategies and " so called safe" practices which are based on professional medical judgement calls, rather than safety studies and in-depth calls to demand increased detailed vaccine safety reporting. Our nation has had limited reporting and studies on vaccine effectiveness for risks in children for centuries. Important forward-looking prospective research on vaccines and infectious diseases occur in other countries at this time, often where the largest populations are, which in short is China.

China is an aggressive drug and vaccine researching country, but the Chinese government also has strict guidelines and an interest in discovering good science. In fact, the United States is most likely in the bottom half of all nations that research vaccines, as our pharmaceutical companies and our educational research system mostly seeks to make a profit from novel vaccines. Regular protective vaccines are mostly an afterthought, left to the government to address. For some implied balance, our government offers a slanted promotional stance freely giving doctors absolute discretion in how they choose to treat patients with no threat of liability. Vaccines are not a regulated drug but an aggressively promoted drug. Doctors are not mandated to administer the vaccines; however, they too are asked to promote vaccines as being part of a political partnership. The push is to mandate other medical professionals, like pharmacist, to administer vaccines and fall victim to any failures of the vaccines in the marketplace, as vaccine injuries are inevitable. Add it all up and vaccines are not what Americans deserve to have as infectious disease treatments under our growing drug laws designed to address drug safety concerns. Enforcement and application of drug and vaccine laws are discretionary with random implementation of rules and applicability of the laws which will always be harmful to citizens.

Vaccine research and development, including experimental uses, have not just grown but have exploded since the Vaccine Act of 1986 was adopted, but vaccine laws and adopted interpretation of the law addressing vaccine injuries have gone nowhere, except downhill. Vaccines are a favorite drug topic among drug researchers and for obvious reasons. Political lobbyists pour in the money to politicians and political parties, and limited liability makes the vaccine drug class very lucrative as a source for investors to profit. Large pharmaceutical companies develop suggestive therapeutic, not protective, vaccine pharmaceutical drugs and use overseas markets to conduct the research to hide clinical findings until they can be crafted and presented for approval by an FDA that is rather slack.

I do not argue vaccine therapeutic science is not interesting, but the science like all vaccine science is not fully developed, and vaccine safety profiles currently take decades to properly develop. Cancer vaccines and other therapeutic vaccines and drugs eagerly pursue a golden payday, when the manufacturers hope to be able to market these vaccines as mass market drugs, when citizens will only have the VICP as an avenue for addressing any novel or therapeutic vaccine drug liability. Even as pharmaceutical manufacturers promote the science of cancer vaccines as being understood or stated as developing a safe profile in clinical trials. Cancer vaccines with specific adjuvants (drugs that increase the activity of the vaccine action to targeted cells) are used to increase effectiveness often also cause nephrotic syndrome. An adverse event thought to be dose or cell function related to increased immune activity. But remember, our highest federal Courts have labelled this as being related to podocytopathy, or specifically not immune-mediated, and our judges do not understand the adverse reaction is a drug-induced adverse reaction, which involves immune system mechanisms and regulating factors, such as ANGPTL4. In fact, Ms. Millman, our VICP special master, believes ANGPTL-4 and the immune system are mutually exclusive closed system processes. Where cells and systems in our body do not work together as a single unit. The federal courts declared the immune system is not involved in nephrotic syndrome patients, as government-paid medical experts wildly proclaimed in the VICP courtroom, in a scramble to cover their other false statements. Our government has declared other nephrology doctors and researchers are wrong, and all parties must understand this new mechanism of causation, called podocytopathy, which could be wrong or partly right, but must be addressed as the current understood mechanism of causation for the medical condition formerly known as nephrotic syndrome as determined by our legal authorities. At least understood until some government expert comes along and changes it at their discretion, or perhaps real science will come into play, and the complete mechanisms will be learned and explained for all citizens to understand.

Yet, the FDA does not care to address many adverse drug reactions that also cause drug-induced nephrotic syndrome, or the need to address such adverse effects that are occurring in many patients. As one high ranking FDA doctor stated, "podo-what", almost like our Ms. Millman in the vaccine court hearing. In the future, the VICP and other courts in our nation will not need to address these misunderstood concern, but can continue to use discretion to choose the suggestive importance of vaccines, over science that relates to adverse events, such as nephrotic syndrome which is predominantly found in children. The VICP and its judicial branch partners push to ignore these risks now for any vaccine approved under normal or emergency (even scarier) use in mass markets, using a slow and delayed system of evaluating adverse events which can take decades. Citizens must understand a vaccine injury is not a vaccine-related injury until our government decides it is a covered injury and listed as an injury in the Vaccine Injury Table. Otherwise, the injury is purely a discretional injury which may or may not be a covered injury by the falsely promised Vaccine Act intent.

At some point vaccine science will catch up and surpass the flawed Vaccine Law, as the science of nature will impose facts that must be understood and addressed as relating to science that is understood and reported, especially as the risks of injury can be further limited with proper protocols and timing-related risk factors being addressed, or as other therapeutic treatments may selectively offset the adverse drug reaction. The time for citizen action under current drug laws is rapidly approaching and may have already passed its end date. The Vaccine Act should be over and done with as a law, as vaccine manufacturers should be mandated to improve its practices of drug safety recording and reporting, with better public reporting that properly addresses valid adverse safety concerns leading to any vaccine-related injuries.

And failing such action by Vaccine Inc (the government and manufacturers), vaccines should rightfully lose their status as a protected drug class by simply ending the Vaccine Act. If the government and manufacturers are honest and open with vaccine facts, then let vaccines prove their worth as safe and effective drugs on a standalone basis as any normal drug would be required to be evaluated by scientists and citizens, or vaccines can simply fade away as a drug class which showed promise for several centuries but failed to deliver on its promise of protection and safety, and certainly are potential failures as a treatment plan or novel therapeutics which could not produce a safe vaccine drug profile for many citizens, beyond the citizens willing to try anything as a matter of informed permission and chosen investigational practices.

As vaccine drug mechanisms work but their adverse drug reactions will never be fully safe or perhaps take centuries to fully understand and manage, or maybe vaccines should be downgraded to being drugs of last resort, and not drugs of first choice as promoted by the government through issuance of recommendations and guidelines. The Vaccine Act failed to deliver on its original enacted legislated promise and cannot be effectively administered to protect all citizens from vaccine injuries, and provides no benefit of promised normalcy for those injured by vaccine-related adverse injuries as promised in the Vaccine Act. In fact, our government's solution generally offers a take-it-or-leave-it, or get nothing, offer to settle a vaccine injury claim, using discretionary understanding of science and a legal process that is outrageously unsound.

The interests of our government and their ongoing support of commercial entities should not supersede the interests of individual citizens. Citizens must address these concerns independently of the government, where our government expresses no interest in addressing vaccine safety concerns with fully informed inclusion of its citizens. Citizens must demand being given full documentation of all vaccine information and important data of recorded adverse events. And medical professionals should be prepared to supply and address the full set of vaccine information records. The current idealistically imagined government-supported information model for advocating and pushing vaccines is an overall failure as a source of these vital records. Citizens cannot accept poor healthcare practices and shady government laws that cut liabilities loose as our accepted medical and drug customary practices. As these actions are a terrible choice for citizens to select from, suggesting should citizens choose bad healthcare, or some healthcare with limited liability which may cause some harm by legislated protected drugs and medical practices. Make your own choice, but do not make the choice for other citizens. They can make their own choices. I suggest the citizens make the choice and not count on the government to provide the facts to make a fully informed and science fact-based consent decision. The vaccine manufacturers are our government's promotional partners, not citizens. They serve us, not the other way around.

Piecemeal information, with a twist of expertise implied but not always correct, is our government's answer to better healthcare. Suggesting for example, a COVID vaccine is over 90+% effective. As currently noted in current studies, and suggesting the only path forward is they will find ways to be more effective, and not less effective, which is again possibly a false promise depending on multiple natural factors beyond our control. Vaccine Inc and the media focus on and promote vaccine effectiveness, and totally forget to discuss reporting of adverse vaccine injuries and adverse events that may or may not have occurred or been reported yet. Remember the lag-time in reporting can take decades.

Having educated and informed citizens with many broad therapeutic choices is my suggested path to better healthcare and a commonsense approach to addressing infectious diseases. Scientific information should be simple and clear, so everyone understands their medical choices. After all, scientific methods of hypothesizing, testing, drawing conclusions and retesting facts are basic and widely understood lessons we learned in science classes. Most citizens know how the scientific methods work; they simply lay trust in the wrong parties to address vaccine injuries.

Should our government be mandated to supply such a transparent and basic forum for citizens to take part in? The answer is yes. Should our government provide training and mandatory continuing education requirements for ALL medical professionals regarding drug safety and laws related to drugs, including vaccines? Again, the answer is yes, and you may be surprised at which medical professionals are not required to do much continuing education, or even expanded educational requirements, that have chosen to offer breaking down into specialized fields of medicine as their answer to better healthcare and public health, which again we know them as being our medical doctors. As with all medical professions, all healthcare decisions are a money issue, and the government sets the standards and regulatory requirements, but rarely enforces them without a big nudge by citizens, and then only act as discretionary actions with favored actions to select political interest groups. You know the interest groups with the most money, who can pay other parties to be the loudest voice on a particular subject matter.

Across the table, the government has been a poor allocator and administrator of good healthcare for many years, lowering regulation of specific drugs, lowering liability for drugs and medical professionals, and other generalized actions which are not the right path to follow and does not lead to better healthcare choices for citizens. Regulation and management through multiple healthcare-related agencies and broad actions promoting a public health system suggested as being in some fashion superior and first class, is simply false. More public money is spent on promoting commercial products and protecting bad actors in healthcare than is spent on basic healthcare for citizens. I know because I have seen it happen in real life. Who manages these regulatory deficiencies? Our government is responsible for oversight in protecting citizens. Can these deficiencies be fixed? Only if citizens demand it, but unaware citizens often do not demand actions to fix such flawed programs and laws. Would the government fix the problems if most of the citizens were to demand they be fixed? Probably not, as the fix is not simple, just as devising a law like the Vaccine Act was not simple but created through lies and promises, to even state nauseatingly the law was to protect our children, where such lies seem to grow and evolve over time, ever since the law was enacted in 1986. Decades of lies are hard to unwind. A simple tweaking of the Vaccine Act is insufficient and would desert citizens impacted by vaccine-related injuries without a long and concerted fight that would most likely be argued based on more lies and false promises.

History tells us authorities in government often give preference to many commercial interests in hopes of helping the government and a few select parties. Public health should not be an area where such discretion and preferences are found to be acceptable to citizens. For historical reference, private-public health partnerships have generally been unsuccessful, often as public funds are used to prop up private interests. The deeper a government becomes involved in the businesses, the more entangled the government becomes involved in the tax and revenue streams. Citizens can argue vaccines are vital to the public's health, but often forget other drugs and treatments are equally as vital. Yet many of these other vital drug classes do not receive the same legal protections or funds for research. How did this problem evolve? Again, under the direction of a few select authorities, who often directed false statements to citizens. Shifting messages of concern (as in 1976) to messages of promotion (as today).

I suggest an open forum is mandated, but it will take a large factional organization of citizens to make it work. Or some may consider it a more radical approach to achieving a solution, which can promote the same message and hopefully result in better future health outcomes. I propose citizens become informed groups of individuals and understand vaccines are not always required as the treatment options for infectious diseases, but are often offered as the simplest and least expensive option used for many decades by our government who prefers not to address the science and medicine, but chooses to promote a cheap and easy promotional drug treatment option for citizens concerned about infectious diseases.

On the horizon, infectious disease medical treatment protocols will surely evolve and address modern infectious outbreaks in a normal and safely evaluated drug development process, but are vaccines part of that future infectious disease treatment plan? Vaccines and the idea of having safe vaccines is undeniably appealing, but not at the cost of individual freedom and choices based on false promises and protections, as our government has actively made a push to coverup harmful vaccine injuries for CENTURIES. In a democracy, we must balance the needs of the individual and the needs of the public. Finding safer and better vaccines will not be mandated until such vaccines must also standup and address safety concerns as all drugs must now address drug safety concerns. Vaccines at one point in history held a valid claim to being a suggestive solution to many infectious diseases as there were no other therapeutic or protective treatment options, and safety concerns were marginalized. Today, vaccines must be held to a higher standard as it is with all drugs, and all drug safety concerns are vital to citizens and to public health.

Currently, vaccines have specialized privileges as a drug class, so as a fair trade for such exclusive privileges, vaccines must also have specialized forums to address vaccine safety concerns, as drug regulators cannot wear two faces acting as the enforcers of drug safety in public forums and hiding facts and safety concerns from citizens behind their backs.

The FDA often fails in that legislated required duty to citizens. The government's self-interests run too deep, for centuries now, starting with the discovery and early promotion of vaccination science and the advent of vaccination policies. The clowns can suggestively run the circus, but the clowns cannot run the science. The Vaccine Act, VICP, FDA, CDC and other government programs are not the forum citizens should look to for answers or solutions about vaccine safety. The VICP however does have a large volume of information which should be openly transparent to the public. And cutting the one-sided government voice that form legal opinions and act as the overriding voice of vaccine science is one path to finding answers. As the government's sole regulator, the FDA, does not address vaccine safety in a public forum. I suggest the clashing of vaccine information from all sides of science and political actions, which will cover vaccine facts from manufacturers, global researchers, and scientists can discard the nonsensical legal opinions formed by legal professionals which have little basis in science or facts. Citizens can address vaccine safety in a united forum and use government resources as steppingstones to better vaccine safety. A sort of, if the government cannot not make vaccines safer for its citizens, the citizens will take action to make the vaccines safer for all citizens by using resources our government and scientists have available right now, which can be a short-term achievable goal.

The longer-term goal for vaccine safety is to liberate vaccines to be independently researched and vaccine injuries to be resolved or vaccines being dropped in favor of other more promising drug therapies. Or perhaps vaccine mechanisms discovered will lead to safer discoveries in a normal path to scientific discovery and could potentially lead to safer infectious drug treatments, without the nonsensical government protection and promotion offered to the single vaccine drug class. But how do we get there? To achieve these goals, first we must take down the Vaccine Act, which will demand an interest by a group of citizens who reject the idea of having choices made for them and reject poor oversight of vaccine injuries. Many citizens already refuse to be vaccinated for various reasons, especially with vaccines that have proven to be problematic and that have causational mechanisms that have been poorly reported and addressed as adverse drug reactions. The unruly call for all citizens to vaccinate and the suggested need for vaccines are largely financially driven statements, which can lead to harmful injuries which will not get properly addressed for many citizens.

But back to fair forums, what do citizens need and citizens demand. I support forums with more transparency and equal access to facts and discovery, especially among citizens injured, and with equal access to disabled citizens, like the vaccine-injured disabled citizens, as required by law. Forums should give equal access to all facts, and not selective facts as decided by a government-designated authority. A vaccine forum should be a singular forum, ran by an independent party who has unrestricted access to all information and agrees to share all information. Add lawyers to the mix, and it becomes an impossible forum for any government to tackle. Our government offers multiple agencies and organizations with multiple interests and opinions that simply do not fit under a one scientific-driven tent-forum model. Public trust and power struggles are conflicting issues, as is money. For many of these reasons, the legislated discretionary model created by the Vaccine Act as its foundation cannot act as the basis for a valid vaccine forum.

As a starting point, I offer **www.VNTY.Health** for a citizen forum as a source for facts for the public to gain access to what are otherwise hidden or not generally available pieces to the vaccine puzzle, except under extraordinary effort by citizens. A place where citizens can get, and give, vaccine facts and details of vaccine injury case reports and studies as reported by scientists, including doctors and researchers, within standards of science and peer review. Our government, and the VICP specifically, does not address global vaccine science, as it relies on the science discovered and supported by our doctors. Science statements being made by American doctors almost exclusively. This odd pairing of interests being founded in historical healthcare and political relationships, and ignoring modern pharmaceutical relationships, which involve global research and discoveries. Science is science as they say all over the world. If a scientist is right or wrong, let the science be proven wrong in a global forum, using scientific methods of validation as proof.

Our government uses shaming tactics to shame those who suggestively "oppose" vaccines or the government's preferred medical partnerships, as in some manner not being scientific, which does not expand our vaccine knowledge relating to vaccine safety but causes scientists to shy away from aggressively addressing these vital safety concerns that harm our citizens. I would like to open up a forum to provide a lot of information, like full disclosure of legal arguments and discussions in the VICP, and vaccine facts reported in case reports and studies, which suggest a different picture from what our government wishes to paint for its citizens about vaccine safety and programs being used to suggest drug safety. And how and where to get more facts and evidence.

Or as many citizens have endured decades of frustration from the current vaccine reporting and vaccine-related injury programs. who want to share their experiences and frustration with other citizens, including the false actions and records of the VICP, ACIP, or any other vaccine-related government agency, where I will try to provide that forum to address vaccine injuries and paths to discoveries. Vaccine safety will not be improved by hiding these facts which are relevant to citizens and must be understood. And real experts in vaccines and vaccine safety will hopefully step forward. My expert in vaccines and immunology is exceptional, but obviously our government has a different view of expertise. I would like a public forum for all citizens to view and evaluate vaccine facts and science, which will not be accomplished overnight, as infectious diseases spark interests but citizen actions must be focused on long-term outcomes and firmly address all individuals' rights.

This action should be viewed as a consumer advocacy forum set up for the express need to inform citizens of facts and ideas, rather than a government-controlled vaccine promotional message board. Thousands of websites currently supply vaccine information, but none provide deeper dives into facts often hidden from the public, or if previously made in public have been removed for various reasons. Where citizens can band together and take collective actions. Vaccine injured citizens often do not have an adequate voice or a vocal advocate, and even if they do, the VICP is not the proper forum for any fair discussion on vaccine-related safety concerns related to causation. The VICP bar lawyers are terrible advocates for their injured clients. The VICP barely functions as an actual court of law but paints a false veneer of being a real court with little valid concern for vaccine injured patients.

Authoritative empathy and scatterbrained opinions do not answer citizen concerns in days of an infectious disease crisis. Authorities cannot claim science will be addressed when little information has not been offered historically to answer citizen concerns. I suggest a forum should discuss the "all or none" arguments. A suggestive are citizens all "in" on vaccines, or all "out" given the lack of liability and concern for safety concerns by our government authorities. A constitutional discussion would mandate citizens should chose to be all out and should reject vaccines without adequate safety profiles as citizens should always have a right to choose and a right to sue for damages, which a jury should decide, not a single government-appointed lawyer. If the argument is, we must protect all citizens, do we select which parts of society warrant the most protection? Children are at limited risk of many infectious diseases and complications. Yet children bear the highest risk of vaccine-related medical complications and injury tied to vaccine adverse responses, along with older citizens with notable medical complications prior to the vaccination. Should older citizens be given more protection, from children who serve as carriers? All citizens should make that choice and these choices should not be decided by government authorities making unproven demands for immediate action.

Any vaccine forum should point citizens to all important and relevant facts, even as many facts are available in the public domain but are scattered using various barriers to prevent easy access. The facts about vaccines should be easily accessible to all interested parties. Drug information is often not easily accessible to all citizens, and the discoveries found through science are slow in being shared in public forums. As some discoveries and cures take decades before citizens are given access to the better treatment options. My personal bias is to focus on understood facts found in relevant and reported science. As citizens can disagree on the importance of scientific discoveries, but forums should allow us to test and retest science observations and drug-induced causation of adverse injuries with peer-reviewed acceptance or rejection of the mechanisms using science as the basis for arguments.

Some vaccine injuries are suggested as unfortunate adverse events impacting a pre-existing medical condition. And if this were the argument, should the Vaccine Act not properly state the law as many injuries which are observed and researched should clearly state an injury is not covered or will be given legal discretion as to what will be determined as fair and just, as the DOJ and special masters have evolved the legal definitions of what is and what is not covered and what is a fair settlement and what injured parties are mandated to take as a "take it leave it, or get nothing" process of settling the injury claim. The current step-by-step processes used in evaluating vaccine injuries by legal professionals create the biggest systemic failure to addressing vaccine injuries and the vaccine-related science.

The Vaccine Act fails our citizens as an unfair and harmful law. For the sake of fair arguments, the Vaccine Act serves no real purpose for citizens, and certainly not for children. All medical professionals should be compelled to know the full Vaccine Act and vaccine-related legal programs and should understand what vaccine-related injuries are and are not covered. Perhaps creating yet another layer of useless medical law knowledge that must be added to the lawyers of useless medical laws that are arbitrarily administered by many government authorities using widely decided discretion. Science addresses adverse vaccine reactions and injuries through scientific research, supplying valid science for citizens to evaluate drug safety standards when addressing vaccines.

Do citizens need proper forums to discuss vaccine concerns? Yes absolutely, and such concerns should be addressed in a far more rapid manner. It should not take decades to address a vaccine concern as it did with GBS. Patients should have a right to address their legal concerns in both state and federal courts before a jury. Judicial discretion and weird decisions would be far more limited if vaccine injury claims were heard by a jury.

Hopefully, you agree and can join the discussion and actions which I hope will change our flawed Vaccine Law. The problems of addressing infectious diseases and drug injuries are equally important, but we cannot neglect one concern in favor of the implied benefit of the other. I suggest we change the slighted concerns about vaccine injuries and make our own statement to reject a law that is harmful to many citizens. As we should also demand justice and proper application of laws as they relate to all citizens.

CHAPTER 12

VNTY

The VACCINE NO THANK YOU Freedom Action Request

A Call for Freedom to Make An Informed Choice and A Public Reply to Our Government.

"I applied my heart to *know wisdom* and to *know madness* and *folly. I perceived that this also* is *but a striving after wind. For in much wisdom* is *much vexation, and he who increases knowledge increases sorrow".* Ecclesiastes 1:17

My final request to citizens is that all citizens should ask a lot of questions, seek out answers, and always make choices that fit your life and lifestyle. Vaccines are absolutely a drug option, and not the only drug of choice in addressing infectious diseases or for use as novel therapies but are simply a drug that must be carefully chosen. A vaccine being a drug choice among many drug alternatives, a choice that belongs to individuals and in the case of children their parents and does not belong to our government. With pressures from many sides, individuals should not feel coerced into being vaccinated with vaccines, like influenza or COVID-19 that are voluntary vaccines. In fact, if a citizen has any questions or is uncomfortable, I suggest citizens use my preferred vaccine declaration to make a sharp response statement. When asked if you would like to be vaccinated, simply state VNTY or Vaccines No Thank You, or simply "no thank you", which you can use as representing your choice to choose what you feel is right in-the-moment as the proper decision for you and your loved ones. I selected the acronym VNTY as a simple message to use and one all citizens should be able to easily remember, and it fits a simple but misunderstood acronym which relates to a misunderstood word, VANITY (without the A or I). If you need a medical-drug professional-approved statement and support for your informed vaccine decision-making right, feel free to select VNTY as your professional referenced vaccine rejection statement. I fully support you with science and testament of false promises to back-up your informed decision.

Why should you choose VNTY as your personal declaration? I would suggest VNTY gives you choices as you can always respectfully ask for more information or walk away, as "no thank you" means "no" in almost every situation. I will provide you additional vaccine information online, but I will state there is little chance I will be recommending either influenza or COVID-19 vaccines as they are voluntary vaccines, and many of the vaccines recommended by our government are not absolutely necessary and certainly do not address adverse vaccine reaction injuries under the Vaccine Act and through the VICP program. Vaccine injuries are complex, and I reject the government's many suggested programs and agencies for addressing adverse drug reactions and vaccine-related injuries. The government's vaccine programs are disgraceful and run by a circus of fools. Whatever faith citizens put in Vaccine Inc's vaccine authorities; I must state are ill-advised acts of civic compliance. Bias and false science are used by our government as reference for nonscientific decisions which harm many individuals. I would reject almost any drug that has this type of false promotional hype with a dreamed-up legal safety net. As a pharmacist, I must understand the mechanisms of action and adverse safety concerns before I can recommend any drug. Vaccines are an aggressively promoted class of drugs with poor safety reporting requirements and an umbrella of disastrous public policies and practices noted throughout history.

All drugs have safety profiles to give the public and medical professionals as an outline of what drugs may lead to adverse drug reactions established through pharmaceutical adverse drug reporting, so citizens will know what the risks of an adverse injury are for any class of drug. As I have stated, many drugs have very poor safety profiles, often initially determined to be acceptable by the FDA, but later determined to be problematic in the first decade or two following initial FDA approval. Many drugs can cause serious adverse medical complications often held back as a concern by manufacturers and the FDA for many years.

Government vaccine research programs have created standard vaccine safety profiles which are often stamped as sufficient using a uniform template and bridged data for comparable protective vaccines. Protective vaccines such as influenza vaccines have a standard government endorsed template, but manufacturers often fail to report numerous adverse vaccine reactions from year-to-year, which has been a standard regulatory practice for more than a century. The manufacturers and government follow the cut-paste and repeat standard for influenza vaccine safety, which may be evaluated retrospectively after several years, or possibly never since the flu vaccine formulation changes almost every year.

A novel vaccine like the COVID-19 vaccine will presumably follow the same standard for a government-endorsed safety template, which will technically take years to develop and evaluate a proper safety profile, and will instead use a shortened emergency protected-use template to serve as a temporary FDA-approved government-endorsed public safety measure. Concerns like GBS or something less understood like nephrotic triggered relapses and serious medical complications that follow, will take decades to address in the current Vaccine Act legal vaccine-injury resolution process, and whether the government even considers it a significant injury related to the vaccine, which will be decided by legal professionals and biased experts paid generously to serve as our government's voice of expertise. These voices of our government do not need to be up-to-date experts, just experts the government can call superior experts in a discretionary decision. The government experts do not need to explain the science or even have a simple discussion on scientific facts, as related to multiple federal drug agencies. The left-hand federal agency does not need to recognize what the right-hand agency is doing as multiple parties do not care to share or review discretionary vaccine decisions as a process of review of science and facts where legal liability and constitutional rights are at stake.

In practice, our government established a centralized purpose of pushing and protecting vaccines as a drug class, with a suggested promoted interest in protecting citizens from an unexpected infectious disease outbreak. The government uses multiple sources of funding and resources to cover the costs of vaccine development and marketing, and the pharmaceutical manufacturers simply switch over manufacturing resources, for a small fee of course, and roll vaccine distribution into established drug distribution channels. And if the need calls for an abrupt switch in manufacturing, our government sweetens the pot, to make things move along faster, as if the Vaccine Act and Vaccine Inc liability protections are not sweet enough incentives to help society.

A novel vaccine with limited clinical data will suggestively roll through the drug review process and receive FDA approval based on an emergency discretionary approval action the public or more likely politicians demand, and manufacturers will disclose some but not all logged adverse events and safety concerns. A vaccine safety profile will be templated by a few experts giving basic data and information for the FDA commissioner to freely approve as a good faith authoritative discretionary decision. Think of it as a medical professional judgement call for everyone, but at least a doctor is making the judgment call, not a lawyer. Everyone crosses their fingers and hope the vaccine will roll out as both safe and effective, and that the FDA will demand post-approval pharmacovigilant reporting be fully vigilant, as normally required but often neglected with vaccine drugs.

If a significant adverse vaccine reaction occurs during testing or in the roll-out to the public, an end to the testing could be immediate or delayed, as in past vaccine injury fiascos. The response by the government has often been noted as being exceedingly slow. However, I am sure we have a bunch of younger Laura Millman wannabes waiting at the ready to step in and save the day for vaccines and vaccine manufacturers, because we cannot have yet another vaccine fiasco, can we? The answer is yes, we can have more vaccine fiascos, and the complications for citizens can be much worse than past fiascos. The Vaccine Act only minimally covers blind faith actions and trust in our government and their unbelievably deceptive promises that they will use science to protect and help vaccine injured patients in exchange for commercial liability protections. We often unconditionally state our trust in God; but everyone else, including our government, needs to step up and prove drug facts using science and evidence. With comparable facts as specified in all drug law clauses that state the requirement for using scientific methodology and documented science to properly evaluate all drug facts, including even the smallest detailed drug facts, which should be available for all citizens to review and assess under their discretion, and must be granted as a right for citizens to make fully informed drug consent decisions .

Vaccine-injured individuals can settle for low settlements or wait years and count on the discretional decision of a nonmedical legal professional to decide what the injury should be worth, take it or leave, all or nothing, and do not ask for multiple medical and financial experts to give science and cost estimates for present and future care of any injured individual. An independent arbitrator will agree with multiple valid professional claim estimates, over that of a paid government amateur life care planner's unverified estimate, almost every time. A disabled or seriously injured child is expensive if carried forward for a lifetime, at least a lot more than I expected as a member of the medical community. Again, I do not set the costs for healthcare, the marketplace sets the costs, which in my son's case Ms. Millman simply failed to accept what the marketplace had set and given as estimates.

And we cannot forget a Department of Justice that will fight injury claims under some devil's advocate narrative to defeat all off-Table claims at all cost, which is an absolutely detrimental expense to an injured patient filing a claim; but not to society as the

DOJ lawyers and officials believe they are in some way serving society by fighting and defeating injured children in a VICP claims process. Is our society evil? Or just Vaccine Inc? I say it is mostly Vaccine Inc as they created and developed the Vaccine Act and its vile legal process for injury claims.

The DOJ and its well-paid medical puppets do not use scientific arguments but use twisted science to reshape a narrative to help the DOJ fulfill their promise to aggressively defeat all off-Table claims. Truth in science does not matter, even where the science and statements do not agree with the government's argument and does not fit the scientific statements of their experts they paid to be on the witness stand as vaccine-related experts. I know now this scientific controversy is endorsed as being logical in vaccine injury arguments. I lived through the arguments and watched them scientifically regress in real life, even overhearing the DOJ changing strategies during a lunch break at trial to "crush my son's case", this being before we played the video that shut their experts up regarding their false facts and science. I never imagined that weird science would be accepted as being "good enough" in any real or suggested court of any type. Let alone a court that is only two steps from the Supreme Court.

All government scientists and medical professionals know vaccines can cause both serious adverse injuries and medical complications. Yet the DOJ and VICP judges want to operate as if the public does not know this fact. The valid medical question is how many adverse events are caused by vaccines, and what can be done to prevent these injures or serious complications from happening again, in future patients. The DOJ and VICP suggest that is not really their problem and science is not their required responsibility to fully address the vaccine injuries. That is the claimant's responsibility, and the special master can without fear of legal repercussions dismiss the argument if it gets too complicated or damaging to the government's experts and defense team. It is no joke, the government's finder of facts can legally stop the discussion of scientific facts in a VICP trial, no excuses needed.

It should be clear at this point vaccine injuries and promoted vaccine programs have been falsely presented to citizens and medical professionals for years. Citizens do not understand the extent of incompetence used by many authorities to deliver incomplete vaccine drug assessments and to make recommendation guidelines. Most citizens do not appreciate the wide range of therapeutic drugs and treatments options available in the drug marketplace today. In-home isolation and treatments by various remote medical setup options make the future of infectious disease treatment plans vastly different than the old-school line-them-up and jab options. A speculative and potentially harmful vaccine should not be suggested as the only drug treatment plan of action.

A doctor that is up-to-date on infectious disease treatments may be the better choice when evaluating treatment options, as therapeutic drug safety profiles will be more fully understood for patients and medical professionals to freely discuss. I do not imply an infectious disease is not meaningful but evaluating infectious disease outbreaks are simply a part of life. A vaccine injury could also be a part of life but could often be preventable with properly addressed drug facts and aid from more drug-trained medical professionals.

Infectious diseases are part of a natural scientific process. Vaccines are man-made drugs designed to mimic natural pathogens. Acts of nature do not carry the same type of liability as actions of man-made drugs, as all drugs administered under some guidance of being safe and effective should be held liable if they are not safe and/or not particularly effective. Citizens have a right to be informed and based on other considerations can decide what plan of treatment options work best for them, whether it be protective or therapeutic.

What you may ask is a safe drug protocol? All approved drugs have understood drug usage guidance and noted adverse complications, but not all drug safety profiles are great or even good. This gives the patient and the medical professionals a valuable point-of-reference to discuss and address use and adverse medical complications that can develop during a treatment plan and where patients must be given information to make informed decisions for their medical state. I have found many instances where our FDA deliberately excludes adverse vaccine reactions from a manufacturer's vaccine reported facts. This is important as it does not give citizens a complete list of serious ADRs. A child is not an adult yet often receives an adult dose, and an elderly person can require a higher dose to get an immune response leading to the development of proper levels of antibodies. Here one could remember my example of cancer vaccines with adjuvants, which increase immune-response aimed at targeting a protective immune-response against the development of cancer cells but also affect immune-responses away from the targeted cells which may lead to other complications like nephrotic syndrome.

A discretionary shortened list of adverse events is the more common standard in FDA vaccine reported adverse event approved literature. Vaccine Inc does not care to devote additional resources to address such adverse concerns, despite the drug laws designed to highlight such vaccine injuries and to address them in a fair and discrete manner which was the intended purpose for the Food, Drug and Cosmetics Act, the Vaccine Act and VICP. I would say the period of substantial negligence and abuse caused by the Vaccine Act should properly lead citizens to demand more vaccine facts and demand information to become more fully aware of adverse vaccine reactions.

The main claim for vaccines being considered safe are many vaccine injuries often resolve through homeostasis, like the clinical body system responses observed when one gets sick then improve and the problems resolve themselves by simply taking a break and resting. A legal definition for a drug injury however falls to a wider definition, which applies to any adverse drug reaction (ADR) as related to any body system injury happening, in any particular, that happens during the window of time a drug is present in the body, and would likely be related to the sequence or cause of the ADR. Drug laws do not state any relevance to whether a drug injury is major or minor, common, or rare adverse events, but that it does occur and that it could be corrected if understood or managed with other treatments options.

Adverse drug reactions often go unreported, as some ADRs are reported in only a small number of cases, and the mechanisms of causation are not fully understood. Science to support the ADR is constantly growing and these adverse drug reactions are being more commonly noted and more narrowly evaluated as to the related mechanisms of causation. Citizens have a right to fully understand what the risks of an adverse drug reaction might be, and what alternative options to treatment or even no treatment might be recommended. It is a citizen's right to be fully informed and to use all drugs at their discretion, not at other parties' discretion.

Everyone does not need to take an antibiotic as a protective treatment simply because a treatable bacterium is spread around a common area and everyone could be infected. There are risks to such aggressive plans, to the patient, to the long-term drug effectiveness, and the possibility the patient may have serious adverse drug reactions. The list of reasons and need to evaluate the need for an antibiotic are long, but patients often skip the antibiotic until they feel worse; but the choice was the individual's choice until hospitalization is required and more advanced antibiotics and drug protocols are required. The adverse drug reactions of the antibiotics are often well-known, and if a patient has an adverse drug reaction, the reaction will often be evaluated by medical professionals and switched to a different antibiotic. These noted risks are well documented for antibiotics.

The mechanisms of action and treatment methods are different relating to vaccines, which are a little more complex to reverse once an adverse vaccine reaction begins that the doctor does not readily identify as a vaccine ADR. Citizens should simply become aware of vaccine risks and concerns and be aware adverse vaccine reactions do occur. Citizens should discuss vaccine use and concerns with the medical professionals, both doctors and pharmacists who are trained to answer vaccine drug questions. And discuss the Vaccine Act and the vaccine programs that function as a liability protection for vaccine manufacturers and vaccine healthcare providers.

Many medical professionals have no concerns in administering, prescribing, recommending, or promoting a vaccine as there is no legal liability for recommending vaccines. The legal liability for all vaccine-related activities and vaccine-related injuries are essentially zero, as in nothing, nil, nada, the big fat not a problem for anyone, except maybe the patient. I find it completely amazing and a common everyday practice to let everyone working in a medical facility, even the door greeters and cashiers readily offer and promote a dangerous drug to everyone, without a thought or concern about any of the vaccine adverse risks and concerns. Vaccine promotions have the highest level of drug discretionary actions imaginable, granted by the Vaccine Act, and promoted through our government, which is an extremely poor dangerous drug policy and are poor professional practices. If that is what people want for public health concern issues, then I guess that is what people will get, but at least ask questions. There are few recommendations in life with that level of release from liability simply by restating a recommendation made by the CDC as recommendations and guidelines being the best policy for all citizens, where the policy is a promotional statement and is not a completely fact-based science statement.

Alternative infectious therapeutic treatment options are available and are becoming more fitting options for most infectious diseases. If you think this is not the current protocols for elite citizens, citizens should go back and check out what drugs were administered to our political leaders who tested positive and were treated for COVID-19 infections. None of the drugs used on our "most valued" citizens were vaccines, in fact none of the authorities made the decision to be enrolled in clinical trials to be COVID-19 vaccine test subjects either. An intelligent and logical citizen can figure it out. Vaccines are not the current best answer for COVID spread or complications, and probably should not be the recommended answer for public health. Competent doctors and pharmacists can recommend treatment plans without a vaccine being needed. Remember a vaccine is not generally used for therapeutic treatment of infections but are used to develop hopefully useful and proper antibodies in a timely and effective fashion, and hopefully without adverse vaccine injuries.

The most common threat to society relating to an infectious disease outbreak is a loss in job productivity, but that problem is not properly addressed, and is mostly exacerbated by illogical actions of our government. What is lowered job productivity without a job? That would be collateral damage inflicted on citizens by poor government management actions, where authorities assume, they know more than its citizens and believes its citizens cannot act responsibly. Better government preparations and utilization of medical professionals would be a safer approach to addressing future infectious disease scenarios. Just do not count on government agencies like the CDC to supply such management and preparations when the government already has many citizens and medical professionals on the vaccine promotional bandwagon.

And finally, the children, who are the least impacted group regarding many infectious diseases and medical complications, but everyone wants to start jabbing them first, labelling them super-spreaders and the cause of the infectious spread among all citizens. The old rule, we must vaccinate the children to protect the adults, for if the children are protected, they will not go into an infectious state and spread the infection. This argument is of course mostly nonsense, but not entirely false. Children often spread diseases, with poor hygiene and other unlearned social practices, but vaccinating children does not ensure eradication or even improved worker productivity, based on statistics used as the primary basis for vaccinating children in the first place, suggesting if the children are vaccinated and everyone else gets vaccinated, productivity will get better among all members of society which is a false statement. These are an old doctor and government leaders' myth used as statements to promote vaccines, which when further examined are false. Children should not be the first "citizens-in-waiting" vaccinated using a novel and mostly untested vaccine, and parents should demand full disclosure of all vaccine injury facts before subjecting their children to potentially serious vaccine injuries.

If traveling to other countries with poor healthcare systems and poor living conditions such travel may call for a need for a vaccine. Bacterial infectious diseases are curable with antibiotics. However, some bacteria are changing, and concerns continue to evolve relating to resistance developing as a problem, and the lack of antibiotics needed to fight these bacterial infections continues to grow as a concern. Consider antibiotics whenever possible, but in a few selected cases vaccines may be the listed drug of last resort required for travel, and may be required as a requirement for entry to the travel destination, which is a discretionary choice to travel made by individuals.

Voluntary vaccines, like COVID-19 and influenza, are not in my recommended vaccine schedule, even as the CDC has recommended annual influenza vaccinations for decades. It is voluntary and should always be voluntary. Especially as our government so poorly watches and reports adverse vaccine complications and injuries. I especial do not want any patients injured knowing the government has not made any attempts to address an ADR as a discretionary action, where evidence and facts were held back from citizens as a discretionary judgement call. Bad judgment calls happen, and bad judgement calls will happen again, and again, and again. History is consistent when it comes to preparing for our government's unsound and discretionary vaccine assessments. My vote is for safety first in selecting my drugs and using strategic pharmaceutical treatment choices to determine the best plan in addressing any medical condition or infectious disease concern.

Parents must remember they are the final decisionmakers for their children. This is an absolute parental decision and cannot be a choice made at another party's discretion. Unless the parents freely give up their rights and offer to let someone else make these important decisions of how to address their child's healthcare needs, such as a doctor or government authority. Sometimes parents are not fully competent but then again sometimes our government is not fully competent. Who do you trust? I trust informed parents to make the right choices for their child. And be wary of vaccinations being offered under blanket prescription orders, or at least get a recommendation from a doctor or pharmacist who has your medical records and knows your medical history. Blind blanket vaccinations are never on my recommendation list as a good medical choice, unless the patient likes to make blind decisions for their healthcare preferred choices. Remember it is a citizen's right to make informed consent decisions, but patients do not have this fully granted right until they are citizens, which occurs when they hit the age of 18. Children are not citizens, and if the parents do not want to be their child's advocate for healthcare needs, our government will be happy to step in and make the recommendations they suggest are needed for your children, generally using broad and blind good faith statements which are also the cheapest option to all parties involved.

So, my highest concern for everyone is that citizens must have a **Freedom to Choose** and to make an informed consent decision about what treatment alternatives best fit their healthcare needs. Medicine is not about discretional logic; it is about natural mechanisms of drugs observed in nature and in the body. The Vaccine Act and our government does not offer quick fixes for adverse vaccine reactions but suggests an eventual fix may address the vaccine injury concern; but it may take a few decades before our drug authorities get around to such evaluations and actions. Vaccine-related injuries are avoidable. Citizens can simply reject the vaccines which are not mandated by law, as it is a citizen's discretionary choice to give consent. Vaccines are imperfect drugs and have long been known to cause adverse vaccine related injuries. No reasonable medical professional is going to argue this drug fact, but instead will want to suggest the protective benefit is a more powerful benefit than the weighted risk of a vaccine injury. I would simply say, "show me the scientific proof" as it relates to me and my health, and "show me the proof there is a valid safety net our government offers" if anything goes wrong and I have a vaccine-related injury.

A complicated discussion will become awkward when confronted with the vaccine choice, and many citizens will simply cave in the moment of making the required last second decision. A citizen will often become captivated by the promotional benefits vaccines suggestively offer, or simply cannot tell a medical professional or cashier, no. My answer to the vaccine question for most vaccines has always been short and sweet. And that is, Vaccines No Thank You, which I invite you to use as your answer as well. I even shortened the answer to an acronym VNTY. Say it twice, if you need to, but you will rarely be asked a third time. Unless of course they do not understand VNTY, which you can show them my book as a referenced starting point for educating the person asking the same stupid question over-and-over again.

I chose VNTY as a shortened version of the word vanity, which is often referenced as someone who is selfish, which is a modern definition. The historical meaning of vanity dates back to early civilization and the importance of thinking about yourself first, and then also thinking about others in order of importance to your life. Surely, citizens frequently have vanity, but it does not mean we do not care for others, we simply care for ourselves first, and then consider the wants of others in order to make fair and sound decisions. If you do not think of yourself or certainly your child, first, there is a good chance you may be pushed to the back relative to everyone else's concerns, which is where individuals often stand in relationship to our government's concerns for citizens.

Vanity embodies a deeper meaning than most citizens consider in the modern usage of the word. The classical translation of vanity works out to have a completely different meaning and not simply being selfish or only caring about oneself. Vanity reflects the individual, which may also signify the importance of friends and family. As noted in the scripture noted at the beginning of this chapter, Ecclesiastes 1:17, vanity relates to an individual's quest for wisdom as an act often suggested as being like chasing the wind. "All is vanity", but what is vanity as noted in Ecclesiastes. For a clearer understanding, the word vanity comes from the Hebrew translation of the word, hevel, which has meaning and reference to mean a "mere breath". Hevel also means breath that has already been spent—so you could say it is a "waste of breath". So why even waste a breath, as it is not worth anyone's time or effort. You can look at other translations and find another word that also means breath and that is ruah. Where ruah means a breath of life. So, vanity can mean both hevel, a waste of breath, and ruah, a breath that gives life, strength, power, and purpose to a personal cause. To have vanity is not pointless and selfish but is a core energy that gives life meaning. In seeking truth and the meaning of life, vanity is essential to all life.

Vanity is also used in classical terms to refer to wind - as a sort of herding of spirits, or perhaps suggested in modern terms - herding a mob of cats. The direction and energy of the wind is often impossible to capture. But if the timing and all things come together, even the impossible is possible. The answers may not come from one individual but may be a collective action of many individuals. VNTY.Health is my individual collection of thoughts and facts captured from my experiences which will hopefully provide positive information to many citizens seeking facts and energy to give hope and life to all vaccine-injured citizens. I do not know if the need for actions is now, or at some juncture in the future. I hope altogether citizens can demand our government take needed actions to protect all citizens both now and in the future.

I hope my simple acronym VNTY will give you vanity to support a cause which I believe is best for most citizens. My vaccine information statement opposes the CDC's widely distributed Vaccine Information Statements given to patients as an information statement related to each vaccine which are in fact oversimplified promotional statements. I do not suggest false solutions or safety and I certainly encourage all citizens to seek facts and truth in science. I do not suggest citizens are foolish individuals that do not understand their drug choices or the implied value of each drug. Or suggest citizens should listen to me for personal healthcare choices. As medical professionals, we look to find answers, and act to spread evidence and facts, so others can seek answers to scientific questions. I offer my respect to those that have spent a lifetime learning their profession, but also understand there is a lot left to be learned in medicine and potentially finding safer vaccine treatment protocols or more likely a need for no vaccines at all.

Medicine entails both clinical medicine and pharmaceutical medicine. Doctors focus on the clinical data. My profession focuses on the drugs. Both professions should be accepted as having expertise in their respective fields. Scientists make discoveries of facts that must be reconciled so they can be learned by all citizens. If you get a chance, tell someone about your vanity, and your support of VNTY. Or simply point them to my website or book. If citizens chose to take no personal action, the choice will often be chosen for us, and that can further complicate our options in the future. VNTY in principle does not require many citizens needing to be heard, but a simple minority faction taking a peaceful action. We understand the choice of foregoing active immunity started by vaccines, which can take weeks to develop and may not provide full protective immunity. We believe in addressing infectious diseases with other therapeutic drug options and strategic conventions as the safest measures to prevent the spread of the disease, and protection from adverse drug reactions which can be harmful to citizens. Citizens alone and in partnership with knowledgeable vaccine medical professionals should aid in deciding a citizen's preferred healthcare choices as related to vaccine science.

Adults making a bad choice and injuring themselves is an everyday event. An adult making a bad choice and injuring a child is unforgivable, and worthy of shaming the parties making such poor choices. The room for error is constrained by a government that does not care to address its responsibility and fails to supply data and facts which can help as they are partners in raising and caring for our children. Children are citizens-in-waiting learning what actions and choices are best. Legal rights regarding care and protection of a child is understood to be equal between parents and the government. Give away a feather and it becomes the government's choice, or the doctor's choice, if you abandon your duty to make informed parental decisions. Parents cannot surrender even a feather in these matters relating to vaccine safety concerns.

Citizens also follow the recommendations of their preferred leaders, rather than being leaders themselves, if only in their small part of the world. Our government proposes a "grand" vaccination experiment to address our current suggested public health crisis, and many citizens simply jump in line waiting for their turn. Some citizens not even asking what the line is for but assuming it must be good. Experimental drug treatment plans often do not turn out as planned, in fact sometimes they turn out extraordinarily bad, like the 1976 Swine Flu Vaccine FIASCO. Doctors and scientists with the kindest intentions often get the science wrong and DO NOT understand mechanisms of adverse vaccine reactions. It does not pay to be on the wrong side of a bad decision by your government, especially in a short window of time to react and change to a corrective course of action.

Early adopters are often the least informed and innocent citizens, who may be misled into thinking they are being vaccinated first because they are in some manner part of the problem, part of a suggested solution or cause for a disease spreading. I state it is simply a bad idea, and one I would reject as a recommendation. I can wait, as I am sure the other therapeutic options are available to treat the infectious diseases and these other drug options will still be available later. Many medical professionals are exceptional skilled evaluators of infectious disease treatment protocols. Why everyone cannot have more useful and safer drug choices is less about medical professionals and more about our healthcare system and the mad scramble our government makes to address public health concerns. So, who should join the Vaccine Inc grand experiment, which may not even be needed or effective by the time it reaches your neighborhood? That is an unevenly debated argument and may be slanted to fit our government's authorities' stated goals and interests. And do not forget, the promise to fix adverse vaccine injuries with the VICP, which is a seriously flawed program for addressing vaccine injuries.

And which neighborhoods should go first in the grand experiment? As some upper income groups will jump in as their professions demand immediate action for implied protections but may not review the safety issues before being vaccinated. If a citizen is in a high-risk profession or a high-income profession, these groups often waive and accept risks and seek a suggested measured protection if possible. Many of these citizens are healthy, and the risk of infection or adverse injury may be minimal in their rush to judgement. I also suggest many middle- and lower-income groups will also be among the first citizens offered vaccines to determine the effectiveness and any safety concerns before distributing the vaccine to other citizens in a large-scaled release. Citizens must remember clinical research testing has often occurred in nations with large numbers of people, and often over a lengthy period of time. The COVID-19 vaccine is being assessed in a limited population and will likely be rolled out to citizens least likely to ask questions. Many citizens will reject the vaccine, and long-term vaccine-related injury concerns may become more obvious. Perhaps becoming understood over decades as mechanisms of a vaccine injury. If you are an early adopter, be wary of the risks of a vaccine injury. As you are welcome to make any decision you feel best exemplifies your immediate health needs but must also accept the impairments of your decision.

My suggested actions do not require a protest or any violence but simple collective actions by factions of concerned citizens worried by our government supplying incomplete adverse vaccine information to citizens. Citizens together can reach out and say VNTY, until we are satisfied vaccines are safer or that we have our legal right to pursue liability for any harms they cause in a normal constitutional process. A VNTY Freedom

Action statement would not be harmful to citizens. It would only require citizens become informed citizens and make good choices. It does not mean citizens will not get sick and develop natural immunity or passive immunity. Social distancing practices and protective gear may help slow down the spread of the disease, but if citizens ignore adverse vaccine reactions, they are also ignoring potentially serious adverse safety concerns. Citizens should make this choice, not government authorities. Our government hides facts and truths which are suggested legal resolutions but ignores longer-term medical concerns. I suggest Vaccine Inc is not playing on a level playing field, which citizens can make better for all citizens by mandating safety first, and by sharing concerns for all citizens through positive expressed actions, by educating and informing other citizens.

There are no guarantees in life, and I can live without guarantees that suggest there is a promise for a vaccine safety net which does not work. In the argument of vaccines versus other therapeutic options, I will always go with the drugs collectively called drugs of first choice with well-documented safety recorded profiles. I address vaccine safety as a higher-level personal concern for all citizens that are at risk of a vaccine injury. Vaccine injuries, like nephrotic syndrome, are not made-up or make-believe medical complications, but have been found to be real concerns, which our government addresses too inadequately as citizen concerns.

Next time you read a CDC Vaccine Information Statement look past the vague and general statements and promotional statements being made by a promotional federal agency. Is the Vaccine Information Statement useful to citizens and is the information patient specific? The CDC does not address individual medical concerns, that decision is left to the doctor to make as a discretionary professional judgement call. A choice which may not fit with your decisions or what you may chose if given more and clearer drug information.

A patient does not have to completely reject vaccines, but simply demand a pause to learn more facts, and can use VNTY as the statement you chose to use to become informed and to learn more about which vaccines you may decide are best for you and your family. Whether you are concerned about a Vaccine Table listed injury, or an orphan poorly documented vaccine injury should not matter, as you simply need to understand the injuries and how they are addressed by all parties for all citizens. So, start asking questions and demanding answers for your informed consent decision which is your right.

Our government's vaccine policy is clear. It is a promotional policy and does not address vaccine safety. The government's voice is an insincere voice relating to vaccine injury concerns as many parties lie, and present false and even perjured statements, and prohibit discussion of facts which are understood or observed in science. Citizens are not given due process, but instead are given false arguments and narratives which are not publicly debated as being related to real science. The important question is, do citizens know these legal claims and settlements favoring vaccines are going on without a public debate and no fair evaluation of science facts, which should be argued in a public forum? The Vaccine Act and VICP are legal actions taken by our government as a means of misleading the public and giving flawed science to citizens which leads to a lot of harm to many individuals.

Citizens often point to rights protected under the constitution and suggest the foundational Rule of Law will correct these injustices. Congress however legislated away one of those individual rights in 1986 and remain committed today to the promotional and legal protection of vaccine manufacturers. Vaccines are above our constitutional rights in many areas, including promoting a commercial entity over an individual's rights without a second thought as to how this affects our freedom and our democracy. We now harken back to the days of admiralty laws with kings and rulers dictating what is mandated for the citizens as they alone decide what is right and what is wrong, and not what citizens choose as being right or wrong. An appointed special master with limited understanding of vaccines and science will decide your fate should you or your loved ones be injured by a vaccine.

I prefer VNTY and Vaccine No Thank You as my ideal statement for personal freedom and my individual right. A firm statement and action that cannot be misunderstood. A call to action that is personal. Not as I have been injured, but someone I love has been injured and disabled for life. I also express deep concern as a medical professional that our government makes choices and deprives citizens of their rights which I have learned and understand as being protected under vaccine drug laws which are currently applied differently as drug laws for a single class of drugs. Our government's actions of creating special and discretionary drug laws for specific classes of drug is not appropriate and must be rejected for future public safety. Not by all citizens, or even most citizens, but simply by citizens that care about justice and truth, and safety for themselves and their families. Vaccines are not a drug with a problem for a few citizens where a vaccine-related injury has caused harm but are problems for all citizens. Ignoring citizen concerns and suggesting we look the other way is never a pathway to answers and solutions and does not lead to a society with better drugs and better healthcare.

If you chose a path of no concerns for vaccines, a path where we do not address vaccine-related injury problems, more serious drug-related issues will ultimately become acceptable results to adverse events in repeating cycles, and will, in almost all cases, result in collateral damage, which will one day be a problem that impacts many citizens directly. A fair warning to all parties to think about before making decisions about such nefarious drug choices. I have thought about my actions and what history has taught us. We must proceed cautiously. Use our minds to make good well-informed decisions. As you may not get a second chance. Our government is the promoter and public campaigner for vaccines, but without all the facts you may not be making the best decision for yourself or your family. I endorse withholding your consent for a vaccine until all facts are presented, understood, and accepted as relating to the level of liability you are willing to accept as satisfactory given an implied benefit the vaccine offers as a form of protection.

Again, there are numerous therapeutics drugs that are always an option in addressing infectious diseases. Vaccines are not the sole drug choice and are not always the best option in addressing an infectious disease concern. I state we must address both safety and effectiveness. All drugs have risks of causing injuries to patients, and people choose to accept those risks every day, often without fully understanding the noted risks for the drug. Many doctors, including Doctor of Pharmacy professionals, help individuals to make informed choices, with facts and professional judgment call opinions using facts and statements suggested as being true from our government and drug manufacturers. Doctors and scientists understand when facts are transparent, honest, and understood, but also know when the facts and science are sly and dishonest as our government has developed a rather underhanded and dishonest voice regarding vaccines. Everyone should know and understand what the vaccine risks and serious adverse concerns are, which must be fully disclosed if requested, so again simply ask for complete facts and information before accepting a vaccine. Or simply reject the vaccine, until you are comfortable with the risks and our pitiful vaccine legal programs.

I fully understand other medical professionals may have a different view of vaccines than I do. Few medical professionals will make deep-dive efforts for research and look for vaccine injury answers even as the risk of injury concerns are often obvious, as these risks are not considered relevant to their patient population or required for legal protection for any bad practice standards. Many follow the government's promoted vaccine schedule and guidance without a second thought. If life were that simple, we would not need doctors and we would not need pharmacists. And if vaccines were as safe and effective as the government suggests, we certainly do not need a VICP or Vaccine Act, or an aggressive Department of Justice single-mindedly fighting to protect vaccine manufacturers.

Citizens should simply decide on drug and healthcare choices based on science. We must broadcast the science and facts, and let citizens share and learn the science through proper educational tools and reported medical literature. Citizens do not need twisted vaccine science designed to fit a false narrative. Our government has practiced twisted science in the art of vaccine drug promotion for many decades now. It is time we demand change, and the actions to mandate such changes are relatively simple. Just say "NO" to voluntary vaccines. VNTY is a proper and fitting resolution to a flawed law which mandates vaccines must stand on their own as dangerous drugs, as our government has set them apart as a specialized and protected drug class. There is no need for citizens to prop-up a flawed and less-than-honest drug class. If citizens want vaccines, even junk and poorly tested vaccines, citizens can make their own choices. If a vaccine is an outstanding drug, it will need no promotion, as the effectiveness and safety will sell itself.

In an age of outlandish drug prices and niche drug development, vaccines are a standout winner for the parties involved in Vaccine Inc. A public "discretionary" ban of vaccines however is warranted, as the government and Vaccine Inc will not listen without strong actions by citizen groups willing to fight for citizens' rights as established under constitutional law. This reciprocal action by citizens to make a choice of no vaccinations without information and fulfilment of promises to protect against injuries as promised in the Vaccine Act would be a reasonable and appropriate decision by citizens.

Foregoing voluntary vaccines is an individual's choice. Foregoing a mandatory vaccine is also a choice but may require more crafted citizen actions to seek exemption. For decades now, citizens have simply allowed the FDA and Vaccine Inc to merrily follow their own discretionary path about vaccine science facts. It is time for citizens to make a collective choice to make informed vaccine decisions. As a democratic society, we must demand facts, demand fairness and a government voice that is fair and accurate, and laws that represent all citizens, especially laws that impact citizens with no voice. May God and citizens show mercy on our children and our disabled citizens.

History has shown us that infectious outbreaks will continue in repeating cycles. And our preparations for many outbreaks will often be insufficient, but it is a natural evolutionary path which must address the many concerns of citizens of all ages and income. The young must not be sacrificed or injured for the old, or the poor for the rich. Individuals can be isolated and quarantined for protection of all citizens, if necessary. Infected citizens will still need medical care, if not in a hospital then certainly at home, with healthcare accessible and provided by families and other healthcare teams overseen by trained and licensed medical professionals. Authorities must address healthcare within their legislative duties. Infectious diseases are always a burden on society, but individuals must find and take proper actions. Authorities cannot and should not be the decisionmakers regarding these personal healthcare actions.

The United States government has suggested the Vaccine Act is a remedy to our citizen concerns as enacted in 1986, but the Vaccine Law and authoritative practices are a failure. Citizens must simply learn more about the Vaccine Act and its deficient vaccine information offshoots. It is time for citizens to correct the failures of our government and compose a statement of our concerns through clear and transparent actions. That statement should be VNTY the next time you are asked, "would you like to be vaccinated?". This deliberate action may take years, or decades, to be received by authorities that have trouble hearing and understanding but will certainly demand government action and discussion which will benefit all citizens. It is a conscientious objection to a flawed promotional drug program created and endorsed by our government. A citizen-based objection that will demand action to fix.

In concision (or conclusion, if you prefer), our government does not properly address vaccine drug safety concerns and science. Our government does not feel a need to address these facts of science. Our government serves the interests of vaccine companies and their personal self-interests. I do not urge you to adopt VNTY for me, but for all citizens. My concerns for vaccine injuries and the methodology and practices of our government, our legal system, and our drug manufacturers and regulators make the decision final for me regarding vaccines such as influenza and COVID-19, and other voluntary vaccines. There may be a proper time in your lifetime to make a statement for your health and for your family's health but do so with facts and science in mind. Science is science, and not selective science as is often applied to vaccines by our government. We must demand facts and demand science or suffer the consequences from our lack of action regarding a fair warning taking into account vaccine risks, adverse events, warnings, and precautionary statements found in vaccine science.

The VNTY Freedom Action Movement is a call for citizens to dissent and demand restoration of vaccine safety to a more normal drug safety standard. All drugs are an individual's choice by natural right and cannot be given alternatively to any other person or our government. Our government enacted a law which ends these rights and harms many citizens using false promises of care and promises to address safety concerns. Vaccines are not fully safe drugs and cannot be granted exemption as safe drugs without constitutional ratification where citizens give up their right to make informed choices. If any citizen is unsure of the need to vaccinate, inquire for answers to your questions, evaluate Vaccine Inc's actions, then simply say VNTY.

Vaccine Inc will eventually get the message but again it may take time. Probably less time than it took Vaccine Inc to recognize injuries from decades ago, as current vaccine-related injury concerns, which is still a work-in-progress, as the injury for GBS is now accepted, but what is a disabled life worth? Not what the Vaccine Act says a disabled life is worth, as a requirement to return an injured citizen's (suggesting children are citizens) life back to as normal of a life as possible. The promised, if not entirely imaginary, resolution plan by our government was big, but the delivery of the pledge now offered is odd and squirrely. Learn the Vaccine Act and vaccine program facts if this statement is not clear. Vaccines and vaccine policies are not a simple tête-à-tête (person-to-person) discussion, but one citizens should take more time to learn through others that have experienced the unabridged version of vaccines as drugs, including vaccine and modern drug laws, proper application of these drug laws, and administrative discretionary actions which are generally harmful.

If you made it this far, I simply must say it is time to say farewell, until we meet again. I say to you, "Vaya con dios, mi amigo. Buen viaje" or "May God be with you, my friend. Have a safe journey". May good health be with you along the way. Visit me anytime at www.VNTY.Health. We can look for answers together. Do not let others steal my message of hope for better drugs and someday perhaps better vaccines with better safety documented for citizens, and a better humanity. Together we can change the world.

This book is dedicated to my son, my wife and family, and to all citizens that are harmed or injured by vaccines. I hope you find peace and happiness in life.

Manufactured by Amazon.ca
Bolton, ON

20435135R00213